CHASING THE INVISIBLE

" . . . unreservedly recommended for both community and academic library Contemporary Health & Medicine collection."

—MIDWEST BOOK REVIEW, Health Medicine Shelf

"This amazing story is about the blending of science, technology and entrepreneurship, guided throughout by unshakable values, to produce life-saving medical technology. In a time of greed-driven business and profit-motivated healthcare systems, this book is an inspiration to everyone who hopes to make a difference in the world. Tom Grogan is one of my personal heroes."

—JOHN M. SMITH, MD, Best-Selling Author of *Women and Doctors*

"Tom Grogan has written a lucid personal saga deftly braided through with medical-detective and garage-startup business thrills that literally pays off with a crucial advance in the fight against cancer. I loved the book and can't wait to see the movie."

—JOE SHARKEY, author of *Above Suspicion*, Former Business Columnist, *New York Times*, Former Assistant National Editor, *Wall Street Journal*

"If anyone can turn the subject of cancer into a page-turner, it's Tom Grogan—and not just because he's an accomplished medical detective. I read this book in awe of Tom's masterful tapestry-weaving skill, his sense of wonder, and his love for medicine, invention, patient care, and adventure. This is the story of Ventana Medical Systems, Inc., a blockbuster company that began as a persistent itch—a need to save time, increase diagnostic accuracy, and track down fiendish cancer cells. Tom features in the book more as storyteller than the star physician, entrepreneur, and good soul that he is. But the real stars of this book are the posse of unsung heroes who collectively produced hundreds of patents to save thousands of patients, rich and poor. For some, this will be a 'Madame Curie' story about selflessly fighting disease through discovery and invention. For me, it's the 'Technology for Good' story we desperately need—about the little company that could. For social impact entrepreneurs, venture capitalists, and students of business, grab this book to learn how to create a social good that happens to make billions of dollars along the way."

—JOANNA BARSH, Director Emerita, McKinsey & Company, and Best-Selling Author of *How Remarkable Women Lead*

"This book is timely and significant! In the life sciences venture capital world, diagnostics has often been overlooked compared to therapeutics. However, with the convergence of artificial intelligence and life sciences, personalized medicine driven by diagnostics is revolutionizing the entire healthcare continuum. Dr. Tom Grogan paints a classic story that strikes the heart of many diagnostic startup entrepreneurs from raising money, building a company, and achieving its breakthrough! When the founder of one of the greatest diagnostic startups writes a book, you arm yourself with a highlighter and pen and read it multiple times."

—VICTOR TONG, Partner of Decheng Capital

"Propelled by his family, his personal heroes, and his own deep passion for improving lives, Dr. Thomas Grogan invented a medical device that changed the way cancer diagnosis had been done for more than a century. His story, and his way of shattering the status quo, is an inspiration to anyone who believes that modern medicine—and motivated people—have the power to change the world. I would like all medical professionals thinking about the future to read *Chasing the Invisible*."

—ATSUSHI OCHIAI, MD, PHD, Director, Exploratory Oncology Research and Clinical Trial Center, National Cancer Center, Tokyo, Japan

"*Chasing the Invisible* reveals medical history: the incredible life-journey of Dr. Thomas Grogan, a young and brilliant pathologist, who left the university with a vision of a medicine-changing instrument. The book contains original 1985 drawings, which he used to translate his ideas of automated immunohistochemistry into reality. Immunohistochemistry has revolutionized pathology and patient care. More than 30 years later, automation of immunohistochemistry can be regarded as a second revolution in pathology. This book shows how Dr. Grogan's ideas gave birth to precision diagnostics in pathology. I think that it is a must read for every pathologist."

—HOLGER MOCH, MD, Chairman, Department of Pathology and Molecular Pathology, University Hospital Zurich, Switzerland; President of the European Society of Pathology

"It is always interesting to learn how we arrive at transformative ideas that go beyond ideas and transform our world. This book describes the journey of Tom Grogan, a pathologist that without question revolutionized his discipline for the betterment of all. The beauty of this book is that not only does Dr. Grogan describe how he came to think of the technology behind Ventana, but also the role of smarts, grit and luck in this successful endeavor. Further, the book gives us a glimpse of what makes an innovator like Dr. Grogan tick through vignettes of his life. The book gives us much to think about and should inspire us all about how wanting to make a difference can lead us to make a difference."

—JOAQUIN RUIZ, Vice President for Innovation; Dean, College of Science, University of Arizona

"Tom Grogan's personal experiences teach all of us that the impact of pathology to medicine is huge. We as pathologists see deeply through a microscope, often delivering difficult news but having the potential to save patients' lives, no matter if they are in Libya or New York. This book is an inspiring, moving lesson for life. Each story holds a message: the power of a positive attitude and generosity; the guiding sense of humanity and discipline; the innate curiosity for science, literature, history and cultures; the willingness to always learn; the creativity; the courage to make a difference; and the great belief that our profession has a mission to help less fortunate people."

—DR. TERESA MARAFIOTI, Professor of Pathology, University College London

"A remarkable story, a loving memoir with elements of a spy thriller, a medical whodunit and a compelling business story."

—D. WICHNER, The Arizona Daily Star

"Great story, well told."

—G. FARR, MD

Chasing the Invisible:

A Doctor's Quest to Abolish the Last
Unseen Cancer Cell

by Thomas Grogan, MD

ISBN 978-1-63393-941-7

Published by

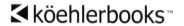 köehlerbooks™

210 60th Street
Virginia Beach, VA 23451
800–435–4811
www.koehlerbooks.com

CHASING *the* INVISIBLE

A DOCTOR'S QUEST TO ABOLISH
THE LAST UNSEEN CANCER CELL

Thomas Grogan, MD

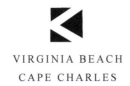

VIRGINIA BEACH
CAPE CHARLES

To my parents, who taught my brother and me

the universe needed improving,

and that we were educated and

capable enough to do it.

Table of Contents

Prologue

A NINETY-YEAR-OLD WOMAN sat attentively in her hospital bed expecting the worst. Indeed, it had been a tiring month-long ordeal beginning with unrelenting splitting headaches. Then the misdiagnosis of a stroke. And next—after transfer to the big city hospital—a mass in her skull discovered on further X-ray scans. Around the bed, a team of oncologists delivered the bad news.

"Undeniably a malignant mass, probably metastatic carcinoma derived from your breast carcinoma ten years ago." There was also a chest mass.

Diplomatically, they gave their recommendations.

"Given the extent of the cancer, and given the toxicity of chemotherapy, and given your age, we want you to consider hospice care. You should consider going peacefully without toxicity. We will see that you receive pain-free, comfortable, supportive care." Advice given, they departed saying, "Let us know when you decide."

With the doctors gone and just me at her bedside, Mom and my eyes locked. Although ninety and weakened by her travail, she remained alert.

"What do you think?"

"First, what do *you* think?" I replied.

"But you're the medical doctor; I need your advice," she pressed.

"I will give it of course, Mom, but you first. *You're* the one who must endure it either way."

"Well, I don't see giving up yet," Mom mused. "After all, they haven't even done a biopsy, and we don't know the nature of the beast. If I am to give in, I would like to know to what. Agreed?"

"Agreed."

"Call the doctors back and let me speak to them," she said.

As the doctors filed in, Mom told them to proceed.

"Bring on the CT-guided biopsy. I'm ready to take whatever you have, but I think we need to know what we're fighting first. So, let's get going; it's been a long month."

"Yes, ma'am," the head oncologist said.

"And one more thing," she continued. "My son here, who is also a doctor, promised to take me to Trinidad to go bird-watching. We are in search of the elusive Trinidad piping guan. So, your mission," she said, pointing a finger at them, "is to get me in shape to go to Trinidad to find the guan!"

"Yes, ma'am," the MD replied.

Thus began the next difficult episode, with another week of scans and biopsies and supportive care. And so it came to be, in that difficult period of being bedridden and pain ridden under the cloud of possible hospice care, Mom and I—with nothing but time on our hands—began to look back in time.

Splitting headaches and eyestrain prevented her from reading or watching TV, so we resorted to storytelling. And Mom had plenty to tell. She had spent sixty-five years as the wife of a US Foreign Service officer, often in high-risk countries in the Middle East and Africa. Truth be told, my father was more than a foreign bureaucrat. He was a CIA operative, leading my family to live clandestinely in the open. We would one day learn Dad had two identities.

Mom had raised three children always with both eyes wide open to the danger, sometimes beginning the evening meal by washing the vegetables in the bathtub with bleach. She knew risk and she knew how to prevail. She knew car bombs and green mambas. She had plenty of tales about riotous mobs and assassination attempts. At times we had literally run for our lives, escaping death. Through it all, Mom remained calm and protective.

My stories of adventure as a young doctor treating malaria patients on remote tropical islands, and of being a professor and medical inventor later in life, seemed no match for the nail-biting adventures Mom had witnessed as the wife of an overseas operative skirting death. All of us could have easily become collateral damage of the Cold War. At the time, she was much more aware of this than we, as I would later learn.

Mom's cascading health zapped her energy and recollection. Details and dates became fuzzy and her voice weak. That meant that the storytelling fell largely to me. Mom was aware of my accomplishments and frustrations as I had shared the broad details of my life's work with her over the decades. But she hadn't heard— and what I had yet to construct—was the full accounting of the dots that connected my professional journey.

I began to recall for her my stories: as an academic medical doctor chasing cancer cures; as a university-based, laboratory-based diagnostician; as an inventor of diagnostic instruments; of my challenges in raising money from venture capitalists and Wall Street; of my founding of a medical device company called Ventana; of the countless legal battles over intellectual property; of my company's acquisition by a Swiss pharmaceutical company, Roche; and of how that event launched our automated instrument around the globe.

Mom knew the plot, and she knew the outcome. But she reveled in my stories just the same. Expressing my life in story form was a repayment for her days as a librarian and a mother reading and telling stories to us and scores of other children. Mom just wanted to settle, even as a child does, in the comfort of a familiar story retold, a real-life story about her son. I sat holding her hand and comforted her as I made the cast of characters appear at her bedside.

And so, the stories flowed, stories about obstacles overcome and of the triumph of human will, stories about heroic deeds and heroes who gathered now in her mind. As they gathered, she delighted in the assembly of like souls, conjuring in my mind this excerpt from an Emily Dickinson poem:

Looking back is best that is left
Or if it be—before—
Retrospection is Prospect's half,
Sometimes, almost more.

From Emily D., our favorite poet, Mom and I learned to appreciate the power of words and how they can inspire. I thank Mom for that. Retelling my stories, and seeing Mom's delight, made me wonder whether others might also find value in them.

1.

Convincing Colonel Gaddafi

OUR REMEMBRANCE OF THE PAST did not start at the beginning. It started with a Libyan doctor whose name lit the flame of my mom's own past adventures in Africa.

Mom's recollection of Dr. Efoud was not random. It reminded us both of the reach and impact of an invention that started in a garage in Arizona. It was an uplifting reminder for both of us at a difficult time.

The young, talented Dr. Efoud reminded Mom of me, the diagnostic pathologist, using the latest chemistry and the microscope to make difficult diagnoses. And Dr. Efoud's interaction with the notorious Colonel Muammar Gaddafi reminded her of the constant task of the diagnostic pathologist to explain to others the hidden inner universe of the chemistry underlying cancer.

Central to this and all the other stories was the story of invention. My invention was an instrument that automated a chemical process known as immunohistochemistry (IHC). It was based on the discovery that a cancer cell can be characterized by biochemical markers from within the cells. With the instrument applying special chemical solutions (reagents) and stains to cancer biopsy tissue placed on a glass microscope slide, a diagnostic pathologist (diagnostician) like Dr. Efoud can identify these markers with a microscope to determine what feeds the cancer cells and what types of chemotherapy can be used to combat it.

Through the automated instrument, the stains reveal the inner workings of cancer cells. They provide a visual picture that illustrates a hidden world. I drew sketches of this molecular world for Mom, sketches that I include in this work to help the reader visualize this obscure cellular universe that, when haywire, can end life.

Dr. Efoud and I first met sipping a cup of tea in Florence, Italy, at the annual European pathology meeting in March 2009. She asked to meet with me on a specific matter related to her medical practice, utilizing my company's automated instruments and tests. We met in the meeting's commercial hall, at the newly constructed Ventana/Roche booth, which featured the recent merger of Ventana's automated, instrument-driven diagnostics with Roche's targeted pharmaceuticals. Ventana's acquisition by the Swiss company had occurred just the year before, in the twentieth year of Ventana's development. The idea was for the automated tests to inform and globalize new targeted cancer therapies, and the medical meeting in Florence was to drive the process of globalization. I was there as the chief medical officer of Ventana, encouraging the use of our new automated tools in diagnosing cancer.

Dr. Efoud and I sat in the booth at a small table. With tea in hand, she came to her specific purpose, which was to bring to my attention two of our employees. She began by calling over our sales and service reps for Roche North Africa to compliment them in front of me. She praised their exceptional service and support, calling them her godsent brothers. She praised their attentiveness and their criticality to her mission. The sales rep and the service engineer graciously accepted her compliments, and I added my congratulations for a job well done. Lingering in the air was a matter of curiosity. I had to ask.

"What is your mission?"

Dr. Efoud explained. "My mission is to improve the lives of all Libyan women afflicted with cancer. My goal is to provide them with better diagnostics and treatment. To do that, to reach *all* of them, I need your tools, your tissue chemistry, and especially your automation."

Covered as she was from head to toe, her intensity could only be read through her eyes and her voice. While soft spoken, of gentle demeanor and thoughtful gaze, she was unmistakably a genuine force of nature. Those eyes revealed a woman who knew that the universe, in general, and Libya in particular, needed improvement— and she was up to the task. She was Madam Curie, Joan of Arc, and Mother Teresa all in one. She was science, service, and sacrifice combined. She was the personification of the Hippocratic oath to care and cure one's patients first, above all else.

"Tell me more," I prodded.

Her story was that of an accomplished diagnostic physician, a pathologist with specialized knowledge of breast cancer. By her description, the lab she had founded and built at the university in Tripoli was world class. She had all the latest and best instruments and testing capabilities. She had three of our top-of-the-line instruments with accessories amounting to nearly half a million dollars in value.

"How did you accomplish all this?"

"From Gaddafi himself," she replied.

"Really?" I was intrigued. "How did that happen?"

"It's a complicated story."

"Please continue," I urged.

"Well," she said, "some years ago, I was running a lab to diagnose breast cancer and inform treatment. We were doing the chemistry of tissue biopsies by hand with a single technician. As it turned out, Gaddafi's sister was one of our patients. Some months after her diagnosis and successful treatment, Gaddafi sent a note expressing his thanks and asking if he could return a favor. He felt an obligation. In a return note, I thanked him and said, 'Yes, how about an audience?'"

Audience granted, her appeal was simple. In order to treat all Libyan women as well as she had treated Gaddafi's sister, she needed the automated equipment, the half a million dollars in technologies. To her surprise, her request was granted, but with a stipulation. She was told to begin small, with a single instrument, and provide proof of its effectiveness.

"Let's see if the seed can produce a tree," Gaddafi challenged.

But what is stipulation to a force of nature? Within weeks, instruments and chemistry in hand, Dr. Efoud was again in audience with Gaddafi. This time it was in the hospital lab, with no regal trappings. This time it was sitting knee-to-knee across a two-headed microscope, looking at a tissue biopsy from a thirty-year-old mother of three with invasive breast cancer.

What Gaddafi saw looking through the microscope is shown here. (See Fig. 1.) Dr. Efoud explained to Gaddafi what they were seeing. The biopsy, now mounted on a glass microscope slide, showed invasive cancer cells. A Ventana gene probe tagged with red dye revealed that a gene known as HER2 was abnormally increased on the cancer cells, resulting in an increase of HER2 protein, tagged with yellow dye.

As Dr. Efoud explained, HER2 was a very powerful driver of cell growth, and the excess HER2 would result in endless, unfettered cancer cell growth, expansion, invasion, and metastasis, which posed a lethal threat to the thirty-year-old patient.

She explained that historically this HER2-driven breast cancer was among the worst types, leading to certain death. As perilous as this had been, it was now a dramatically improved circumstance since Roche/Genentech had developed a powerful anti-HER2 therapeutic antibody known as Herceptin˚. This drug blocked and shut down the HER2 growth receptor, causing the cancer cell's demise. For the thirty-year-old Libyan patient, a cure was very likely.

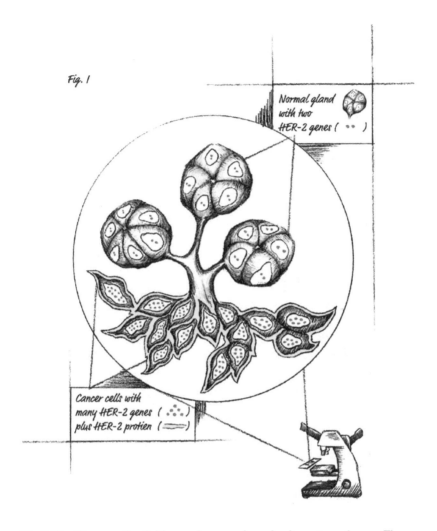

Fig.1. The Libyan patient's biopsy shows an invasive breast carcinoma. There are three normal breast glands (blue) arranged in round and regular clusters like plump grapes. Below them are scattered irregularly-shaped, raisin-like cancer cells (yellow), which are no longer contained within the gland but invading the adjacent tissue. The normal breast cells have the expected (physiologic) two HER2 genes (red)—one from mother and one from father. The cancer cells have an abnormally (pathologically) increased number of HER2 genes (red), and an excess of HER2 protein (yellow) on the cell surface. The cancer cells are clearly altered morphologically (in physical form), phenotypically (in protein status), and genetically (in gene status).

Finally, Dr. Efoud emphasized that with her new automated Ventana/Roche instrument and chemistries, she could now do what no one could do by hand. Thanks to the precision and control of automation, she could combine the gene and protein tests to definitively identify a target of therapy.

What Gaddafi learned that day convinced him, and he removed the stipulation. The money to provide for all Libyan women was willingly given. Mission accomplished. Well, nearly; at least the means were at hand. It was at that moment, sitting with Dr. Efoud for tea, that two thoughts emerged for me.

The first, that sitting before me in all humility, only seeking to thank others, was a saintly person. A person who brought hope and good to the world. A person unconstrained by dire circumstances. A person who belonged in the assembly of the like souls Mom revered.

Second, I thought of Gaddafi on that day, as a powerful man, as a brutal dictator and a bearer of force, a man who was party to the Lockerbie bombing—and how he must have felt the force of her knowledge, her humility, her persuasion. He must have, sitting at the microscope, felt the power of making the invisible visible, of making the lethal treatable, even curable. Given his subsequent beneficence, he must have felt compassion for his people, brought out by hers.

The retelling of this story six years later in a dimly lit hospital room rekindled in both Mom and me the reassurance that saintly persons may still prevail, and even a dictator may feel compassion.

In Mom's remembrance of her past adventures in Africa, she recalled that Gaddafi and his agents were part of our family history. She was roused to tell of Dad's assignment to Timbuktu, Mali, from home in Liberia. He was there on a covert mission as a CIA operative to re-establish contact with an agent who had gone silent, cause unknown.

It was the late 1960s and contact with the missing agent was critical as he was the eyes and ears following Gaddafi's incursion into the sub-Saharan Sahel. With contact broken, the CIA was blind to his nefariousness.

The unusual part was that Dad, along with his supporting cast, traveled to Timbuktu on the last stretch by camel in a caravan, as there were no functional roads, no trains, and no planes.

Almost as remarkable was the fact that it was only that night, by her hospital bedside, that I first heard this story of Dad's exploits in Timbuktu. But these long-hidden memories come with the territory when you grow up in a family engaged in clandestine affairs. Secrets are not secrets if told to another. For true deception to go unnoticed, it must be unspoken.

The recollection of Dad's exploits in Mali invigorated Mom. When you're marooned in a bed for a month, a bit of adventure relived is an elixir. A tonic to sustain the fight.

2.

Finding our Everest

HAVING BEGUN IN THE MIDDLE of this fifty-year tale with recollections of those exotic Libyan events, Mom felt invigorated. She asked if we could go back to the beginning.

"Tell me about how you came to the need to invent."

Inventions are not born out of comfort and satisfaction. They are not born out of a sense of accomplishment or a sense of well-being. They are born out of thwarted accomplishment, a sense of disquietude, or an unmet need.

When I came to the medical school at the University of Arizona in 1979 as a new assistant professor, I wasn't thinking about inventing. I felt a great sense of satisfaction and achievement. I had earned a good position, and I anticipated further accomplishment in my field of clinical and anatomic pathology.

I came bearing intellectual gifts. I was straight from training in the lab of a world-famous professor at Stanford, and he had armed me with the latest technology: monoclonal antibodies. As I learned from him, when the newly developed monoclonal antibodies had dyes attached, we could splash them on tissue biopsies, and then we could see the cellular chemistry with a microscope. Done by hand, the process was very similar to developing a photographic image.

Looking in the microscope, you could see for the first time the inner workings of cells. You could now identify individual cancer cells and determine what made each one tick. And from that, what type of chemotherapy might be used to successfully treat it. Every new probe we used led to new images and findings. It felt a lot like astronomy a hundred years ago when, for example, Pluto was discovered on a developed photographic plate. Now, instead of looking out with a telescope, we were looking into an inner universe with a microscope. For an academic, it was a field day.

Every day brought new discoveries, and every month we published new findings. Like Darwin in the Galapagos, everything seen was previously unseen. His geography was oceanic and mine was anatomic, but circumnavigate we did. From this there was no discomfort, no dissatisfaction, no thwarted accomplishment, no disquietude. There was therefore no need to invent.

The need to invent began first with others close to me: Catherine Rangel, my assistant, and Dr. Tom Miller, my oncologist colleague.

Catherine was the head technician in my lab, with twelve years of experience as a histologist. She and the other techs, Yvette Fruitiger and Lynne Richter, handled all the tissue coming from the hospital and the clinics. They snap-froze the biopsy tissue, then glued the tissue onto glass slides and stained them with dye-labeled antibodies in the process known as immunohistochemistry (IHC), which then allowed diagnosis by microscopy. Catherine also directed the graduate students and residents in the lab, overseeing what we called the *bucket brigade,* which was the daily all-consuming measuring and mixing of the more than fifteen solutions and solvents needed to stain slides by IHC. The process filled the working day of all three technicians. It entailed the formulation of liters of solutions and an assembly line of glass slides, each with a sliver of tissue from a patient biopsy. There was frequent last-minute mixing of volatile, short-lived chemicals. Some of the chemicals were highly carcinogenic, requiring a protective gown, mask and cap while cramped in a protective air-controlled glass hood. The just-mixed chemicals were then laboriously hand-applied with a pipette one slide at a time. New reagents were being added and washed off the slides every fifteen to thirty minutes. As several patients were being studied at once, each with their own formulation, it was an endless mental exercise in combinatorial optimization. Further adding to the chaos, there was a cacophony of lab timers (equivalent to high-pitched alarm clocks) going off every ten minutes to signal the need to add or remove reagents. This auditory assault was compounded by the phone ringing with impatient MDs calling for results, and as every tech knew, ignoring those phone calls could be followed by the physical appearance of a pissed-off surgeon. The workplace was unequivocally toxic, clamorous, demanding, unforgiving, high pressure, laborious, tedious and at times outright hostile. In the hospital, much was at stake. All relied on speedy results. For the techs it required Olympic fortitude, mechanical adeptness and mental toughness to deliver timely answers and make it through each day. Oddly, the pathologists were not so troubled as they sat in the comfortable office down the hall. In retrospect, it is not a surprise that the impetus for automation came first from the techs and not the MDs.

One year into her job, under those difficult conditions, my technical assistant, Catherine, was to become the mother of invention. She was the first one to seek to change the work environment. Besides the techs' needs, she identified the critical need of the patient for a speedy diagnosis. She did this through her everyday experience in the lab and by personal connection to patients in the hospital.

Besides running the lab, supervising the trainees, and doing all the chemistry by hand, Catherine was given another demanding assignment. She was charged with going to the clinics and operating suites to pick up the tissue biopsies. I had imposed this burden on Catherine through the simple act of posting signs in the clinics and operating suites. The signs read, "Before you take it out, call the Grogan lab to handle the tissue."

That sign had an intentional consequence, and an unintentional consequence. As intended, it meant we always had fresh tissue, which we then snap-froze and preserved for study. The pristine preserved tissues ensured that we had biologically sound results, which over twenty-five years ensured many thousands of accurate diagnoses and more than 250 scientific papers. That was intentional.

But the unintentional consequence was to be of far greater magnitude. It spawned an invention and eventually a company—Ventana.

When called, Catherine would arrive promptly in the patient's room fifteen to twenty minutes before a biopsy in order to be ready for the doctor. Then came the magical part. In the twenty minutes it took to complete the task, Catherine had, by virtue of her engaging personality, made a friend for life of the patient. And so, the unintentional continued.

I recall one day at 7 p.m. when I was ready to leave the hospital. It was dark and I was tired. At the lab door, I was stopped in my tracks. In a booming voice, Catherine demanded, "Where are you going?"

"Home," I replied.

"Why?" she asked.

"Because I'm tired, it's dark outside, and it's dinner time."

"Not so fast," she said. "I told Mrs. Jones we would have results for her first thing in the morning. Dinner can wait. The patient can't."

"Really," I balked. "And who is Mrs. Jones?"

"She's Dr. Miller's patient, whose biopsy I have been working on since yesterday, and I need you to read the slides now. She has been told it is probably breast cancer. She's terrified, and I told her we would get her results ASAP. She is a thirty-year-old fifth-grade teacher with two kids and a husband, and she is sitting on pins and needles. Dr. G, we must help her now before she spends all weekend in a panic."

I read the slides that night, and Dr. Miller was in the lab early the next morning to review them. As Mrs. Jones feared, it was an invasive breast carcinoma; that was the bad news. But as Dr. Miller and I looked in the scope, we saw the good news (see Fig. 2). The tumor was a small, estrogen receptor–positive (ER-positive), hormonally driven cancer. So, presuming her lymph nodes and scans were negative, the treatments consisting of lumpectomy and targeted anti-ER therapy (Tamoxifen) could very likely cure her. Reassuringly, over the past twenty years the mortality of breast cancer had decreased by nearly 25 percent, largely due to early detection, better scans, and anti-ER (estrogen) therapy.

Dr. Miller was pleased. When he talked to the patient, he would have a definitive diagnosis, a mechanism of disease, and a target for therapy. As he well understood, the bad news would be mitigated with knowledge of a likely curative therapy. So armed, he thanked us for our promptness and ended with a plea. "I want you to do this for every one of my patients."

I paused and replied, "Sorry. Not possible."

"But you just did Mrs. Jones so promptly," he pressed.

"It took us two days," I said, "and you have a clinic with fifty patients. It's just a few of us, and not enough daylight."

With Dr. Miller leaving, I found Catherine glaring at me. "You said no!" she huffed.

I pointed out how hard the techs were working to produce results manually. It was very laborious, tiring, and unsustainable. We lacked the tools to deliver to everyone, every day. We lacked automation. We were plowing with a horse and needed a tractor. Our chemistry by hand was like photography before the Brownie automatic camera and Kodak film. So, I concluded, "No matter how much we want to, we cannot give every patient answers quickly."

Without hesitation, Catherine shot back, "Then build something that can!" That refrain became a daily mantra.

And so, Catherine came to find our disquietude. She found, by connection with patients, their hidden need. She established our need to invent with her call to action. *Build something that can.*

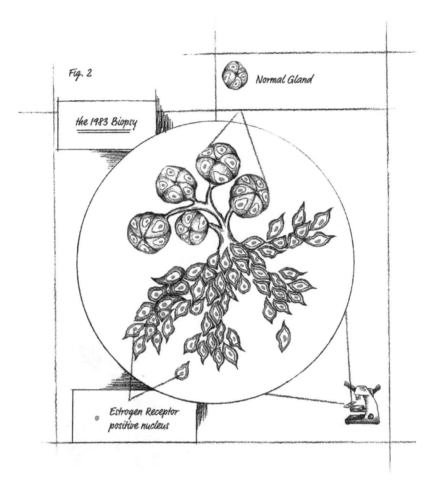

Fig. 2. Mrs. Jones's biopsy shows an invasive breast carcinoma positive for (expressing) estrogen receptors. There are five normal breast glands arranged in round and regular clusters like plump grapes. Below them are scattered irregularly-shaped, raisin-like cancer cells invading the surrounding tissue. Both the normal cells and the cancer cells are positive for estrogen receptors (red) in the cell nuclei. This indicates that both the normal cells and the cancer cells are hormonally driven to grow and would die with an anti-estrogen drug.

The seed was planted. The quest was on. The imperative of the lab would be the patient—not the publication. The spell of splendid academic isolation was broken. Catherine's voice kept echoing, *"If you can't, then build something that can."* And so Catherine and I had discovered our *why*—because Mrs. Jones was waiting, because all the other Mrs. Joneses were waiting. Like Edmund and Norgay, we had found our Everest.

It's funny how a mountain calls you to the top without ever asking if you are otherwise occupied.

The night of that telling, Catherine fit snugly at Mom's bedside as a rightful member of the assembly of like souls, and as always, she brought us great cheer.

Within a week, the quest intensified. The occasion was the return of Dr. Tom Miller to the lab to view Mrs. Jones's lumpectomy specimen and her lymph nodes. As we looked in the scope together, the news was good. The margins (areas around the tumor) were cancer free and lymph-node negative. He added that MRI and CT scans were also negative for cancer.

With Catherine standing nearby, he explained that cure was now very likely as the mass was small, the margins and lymph nodes were free of cancer, all scans were negative, and the tumor was, indeed, hormonally driven. She would take daily doses of Tamoxifen, for five years. Catherine—ever mindful of tending her flock of patients—was pleased to hear the news, and then, as was her wont, she turned quizzical.

Her brow was furrowed, and her brain was abuzz when she asked Dr. Miller, "If the margins are free, and the nodes and scans are negative with no evidence of disease, why are you treating her with a drug? What's the sense of treating something that is no longer there? You're treating the invisible. Why put her through the pain and expense of further therapy when she is already cured? Couldn't the drug harm her? Why do it for five years? And how do you know it's working if you can't see what you're treating?"

Then, not waiting for answers, she turned to me and asked, "If she's disease free, why did we do the chemistry on her tissue? Why do the IHC when there's nothing left?"

Dr. Miller spoke up. "Disease free and cured are not necessarily the same. She could be free of the disease now, but it could recur in the future, despite the surgery. To cure her, we have to kill every last cancer cell, including those we can't see, because it only takes one for it to persist and recur."

He continued. "It's like killing cockroaches; you're not finished just because you have killed the ones you see. You have to go on with a systemic chemical treatment of the whole house to get every last one. Then you have to repeat the treatment because the eggs lie dormant and come to life days or weeks later. It's the same with cancer cells. That last unseen cancer cell can shut itself down, put the dimmer on and go dormant, returning and growing days or months later.

"Hence the need to keep Mrs. Jones on Tamoxifen for five years. That's what it takes to kill the last unseen cell, the last dormant egg. That is what it takes to cure someone. So, yes, Catherine, you're right. To get that last unseen cell, to cure the patient, we must chase the invisible. And as for performing immunohistochemistry on the biopsy, that is critical to identifying in the individual cancer cells the nature of the beast, the mechanism of disease, the driving force and the cancer cell's vulnerabilities. So, for Mrs. Jones, we know her tumor is ER-driven and therefore our anti-ER drug should destroy the last unseen cell. Her treatment is targeted and informed by the chemistry that you all do."

Taking it all in, Catherine had one more question for us. "Is this true of every cancer?"

"Ultimately, yes," Dr. Miller replied. "This one happens to be hormonally driven, but there are hundreds of other driver events. That is why the testing must be so elaborate. We go until we find the nature of the beast, till we find a driver event, till we find its vulnerabilities and the target for therapy."

"So, it's not just that every patient needs this, but they need many more tests than we're doing today?" Catherine asked. "I guess that settles it. We simply can't keep up by doing the chemistry by hand. As I said last week, it's time to build something that will."

And so it came to be that Dr. Miller added another layer of intensity to the quest. Catherine had brought us the patient's need, and Dr. Miller brought us the physician's need to know the diagnosis, to know what made the cancer cell tick, to know the mechanism of disease, and to find a target for therapy. He was driven by Hippocrates's charge to physicians to attend to the care and cure of their patients.

Dr. Miller had added another *why* to our equation. There was already Catherine's why—because the patient needs answers. Now we had Dr. Miller's why—because the doctor needs answers to chase the invisible threat to life.

Mom followed this part of the story closely. She was keen on the thinking of oncologists as she was on her third bout of cancer, having endured numerous rounds of chemotherapy and radiotherapy. Because she had heard Dr. Miller speak before of "chasing the invisible," she understood his concept well. She also understood it was, at that time in the 1980s, new to medicine to move all that chemotherapy up front (so-called adjuvant chemotherapy) when the patient was scan-negative after surgery and radiotherapy.

Having been around Dr. Miller in those early pioneering days, Mom recollected that his aggressive up-front chemo approach was at first hotly contested.

As she recalled, "Wasn't he shouted down publicly by some of his fellow oncologists?"

"He was—I remember well," I replied. Then I recalled a contentious medical meeting of the American Society of Clinical

Oncologists (ASCO) in Chicago in 1979. At that annual ASCO meeting, Dr. Miller presented his pilot study of twenty patients with localized malignant lymphoma who were first treated by surgical resection of the tumor and then, in spite of being scan-negative, were treated with add-on (adjuvant) chemotherapy followed by monthly maintenance chemo.

Historically, these scan-negative patients would receive—at most—local radiotherapy to the disease site. However, despite both surgery and radiotherapy, relapses were common. Since these recurrences were often at distant sites in the body, Dr. Miller reasoned that to prevent distance recurrences and cure them, a systemic drug treatment, not a local one (radiotherapy), was required. His measurable end point was a reduction in recurrences, which was beginning to show in his twenty patients. But all this add-on chemotherapy, including toxic drugs like Adriamycin˙—which could cause cardiac damage—was new to medicine.

His study was soon to publish in a top journal, *The Lancet* (Miller and Jones pp. 358-60), and eventually, with more patients included, it was published in the *New England Journal of Medicine* (Miller pp. 21-26) and was to become the new required standard of care. That definitive NEJM study took more than a decade to complete, as it was necessary to "prove a negative"—as in, recurrences that never occurred. Calling the patients "cured" required years of follow-up.

But all of that was years ahead, and on that fateful day in Chicago, before several thousand oncologists, there was vociferous criticism of Dr. Miller's unprecedented aggressive approach.

When he finished presenting his data, they lined up at the microphone by the dozens to criticize, saying things like:

"This is malpractice."

"This is unnecessary overtreatment of a patient who might already be cured."

"This is adding the risk of chemotherapy-related complications."

"This is putting the patient through toxic hell!"

"This will cost us all millions of research dollars trying to prove a negative."

"This will require a double-blind clinical trial involving hundreds of patients and will cost a fortune."

"This is a dangerous approach without precedent."

Dr. Miller took on the challengers one at a time, reminding the audience that a similar approach, employed by Dr. Emil Freireich of MD Anderson Hospital, proved curative in acute leukemia. Why not other cancers?

But the protests continued. Finally came the most vocal of them all—a prominent academic professor, known to all in the room, who condemned Miller for risking so much while stupidly "chasing the invisible."

While it seemed like the final definitive dismissal by an influential authority, Dr. Miller's response was immediate and unexpectedly buoyant.

"Thank you for putting it that way," he said. "You are absolutely right. To cure all patients, we must *chase the invisible*. You have given me my mantra."

And so, it was on that fateful day, before thousands, that our mantra was born—*To cure, you must chase the invisible.*

It's funny how criticisms, as unpleasant as they may be, can crystalize and galvanize a movement. And it's funny how a ninety-year-old ailing woman could hold a crystal-clear recollection of distant events.

The call from Catherine and Dr. Miller to invent, to create new tools, and to develop an automated instrument was strong and persistent, but it was after all just an aspiration, however compelling.

As the head of the lab and the leader of our intellectual enterprise, it fell to me to go beyond aspiration and to deliver. It was one thing to imagine a solution to a problem, but another to execute that solution.

As I was still—in the early 1980s—just an assistant professor without tenure and without job security, why risk a promising, productive academic career? As an academic I was expected to publish peer-reviewed scientific papers and to write proposals for government grants to pay for the techs' salaries, our lab supplies and the department's lab space and utilities. By the usual academic standards, it was publish or perish. There would be no credit for creating an automated instrument; that was industry, not academia. The monastery had rules. It was likely career ending if I embarked on a diversionary journey into business and industry, where I had no schooling whatsoever.

That lack of savvy being understood, why would I divide the attention of the lab, the graduate students, and the resident trainees? Why pursue naively what you could otherwise pursue knowledgeably? Why leave *terra firma* for *terra incognita* over uncharted water? Why risk being adrift on strong currents that may take you to un-wadeable depths?

And so, to be a responsible leader I had to weigh not only the aspiration to invent, but the risks to all of us. It was at this juncture of uncertainty that my own call to invent gained conviction.

As we began to develop more and more tests by hand out of the Grogan Lab, and as the chemistry on each biopsy done became more elaborate, I began to influence the hospital practice beyond Dr. Miller. I began to systemically change the mindset of our physicians at the University of Arizona Medical Center. Our faculty and residents numbering over 250 noticed a new level of diagnostic certainty. In the faculty dining room, the talk was of this new approach that changed diagnoses and treatment.

There was the ten-year-old boy said to have a cancer of the tonsils whose planned radiotherapy and chemo were halted when we proved by our immunohistochemistry (IHC) and in-situ hybridization (ISH) that he had, in fact, a bad case of infectious mononucleosis. He subsequently recovered without chemo, having received supportive airway care and a liberal dose of lollipops—that old standard of pediatric care relevant to self-limited disease.

There was the fifty-six-year-old woman said to have a lymphoblastic lymphoma whose chemotherapy was stopped, having proved by IHC that it was a benign thymoma cured by simple surgical excision.

There was the forty-two-year-old in a coma said to have meningitis unresponsive to antibiotics whom we proved, upon doing IHC, to have instead a rare CD30-positive form of cerebral lymphoma, which was found to be chemo sensitive. Word of her transfer from the infectious disease ward to the oncology ward, and her subsequent recovery from the coma on chemotherapy, quickly spread throughout the hospital.

This is how every difficult, obscure medical case began to come our way. Every lump and bump needed our IHC chemistry and my attention. Like Catherine and Dr. Miller, I was inundated and needed automation to assist.

There was one other compounding factor that heightened my need to invent—what you might call publicity. As you may know, MDs are not permitted to advertise, at least not in the media. But by word of mouth, MDs in the surrounding hospitals sought our services and my opinion. This growing circle of need was enhanced by my chief, Dr. Jack Layton, who strongly encouraged me to present my game-changing IHC cases at medical forums.

Jack, the chairman of pathology at the UA medical center and a well-known academic pathologist on the national scene, was excited by our clinical success and began signing me up for every available medical meeting, from the local monthly Tucson Pathology Society, to the Arizona State Annual Pathology Society, to similar meetings in New Mexico, Utah, Nevada, Idaho and Oregon. My format involved sending participants a box of glass slides containing the diagnostic tissue biopsy of ten or so patients. After all mailed in their diagnoses, we would meet for a daylong continuing-education meeting. I would then reveal the IHC findings for each case, which often had the effect of either confirming a difficult diagnosis or changing a debated diagnosis with greater clarity. This format, a long-standing tradition in medicine of learning from your patients, demonstrated to medical practitioners how tissue chemistry by IHC was improving diagnosis. On this basis, the floodgates of consultation opened.

Five years on, in 1984, I had a consultation practice based on IHC that extended from Los Angeles to Dallas, from Salt Lake City to Mexico City.

The addition of Mexican consults came after I presented at a joint meeting of the Arizona and Hermosillo, Mexico, pathologists. I presented the case of an eight-year-old boy scheduled for amputation at the knee due to a malignant bone tumor in his right tibia. We were sent the tissue block to confirm the diagnosis, but our IHC showed it was in fact a benign S100-positive Langerhans cell tumor. The amputation was canceled, and radiotherapy proved successful. Soon, tissue blocks from Mexico arrived weekly for further study.

By the end of 1984, I was coming to the lab each morning to find a mail sack with five to ten tissue blocks and requests for consultations. And so, like Catherine and Dr. Miller, I now needed automation to handle the growing number and sophistication of consults.

In retrospect, Catherine and Dr. Miller had started this quest to automate by connecting us to the needs of the individual patients who were at our own hospital. I then added another compounding need—the need to go beyond us and our hospital to others. The need was to improve medicine everywhere. The need was universal.

3.

Magellan and Me

MOM KNEW MY ASSISTANT, CATHERINE, and Dr. Miller personally, and she understood how important they were in spurring me on. Thinking back to those early days, she asked me to remind her how I went from leprosy to cancer, from internal medicine to pathology. She wanted to hear about the circuitous route I traveled over the course of my career, and about the decisions that guided my unorthodox path. And so I began to retrace my earliest steps.

My journey to that pivotal juncture in 1984 commenced seventeen years prior when I went from neophyte medical student to becoming an expert in my field of hematopathology (blood diseases). This entailed four years as a medical student at the George Washington School of Medicine, a year as an intern in internal medicine, four years of residency in pathology in San Francisco, two years running the hematology lab at Walter Reed Army Hospital, a year of fellowships in hematopathology at Stanford, and five years as a young assistant professor at the University of Arizona.

Thinking back, there were several transformative events that brought me first to the field of pathology. The first occurred on a remote island in the Philippines known as Cebu. My journey there began in 1970, about 450 years after the Portuguese navigator, Ferdinand Magellan, made his landmark journey there.

As it turned out, neither Magellan nor I expected our travels to Cebu to turn out as they did. Magellan unexpectedly ended his journey there in 1521 at the point of a spear, and I unexpectedly began mine in 1970 at a leprosarium.

That summer, as a junior medical student on a National Institutes of Health (NIH) traineeship grant, I had chosen to work at the Eversley Childs Leprosarium on the island. My intention was to study tropical medicine, to imagine myself as Albert Schweitzer, pith helmet and all. With my wife, Cande, at my side (she was off from teaching first grade that summer) we were given a full introduction to the world of tropical ailments.

In addition to my duties at the leprosarium, we traveled weekly with the Philippine public health physicians and nurses. Typically, we took a light plane to one of the hundreds of islands nearby. We would set up a medical station while the villagers lined up for exams. Although just a junior medical student, I was deputized as one of the examining MDs. In those lines of villagers that summer, I got a crash course in the full range of tropical diseases—from malaria to yaws, from schistosomiasis (caused by parasitic worms) to elephantiasis, from tetanus to opisthotonos (tetanus-related paralysis), from dog bites to rabies, from typhus to typhoid. The ravages of infectious diseases were everywhere. But we came to the rescue. We were armed with a full pharmacologic armamentarium, and our diagnoses and treatments were immediate.

To a US medical student accustomed to being in line behind the attending, the resident, and the intern physician, this was thrilling. I witnessed things even my professors back home had never seen. It reaffirmed my commitment to go into internal medicine.

In recounting this experience to Mom, several dramatic events stood out in my mind from our time with the public health group. There was the call to go to Mactan Island, right next to Cebu, with word of a typhoid epidemic. You might call it Magellan's revenge, as it was the very place where he was killed in 1521. In that July of 1970, a whole village came down with typhoid-caused septicemia/fever, and while medical care in the Philippines was then free, medications were not. So, I spent part of my stipend from my NIH traineeship and bought $250 worth of chloramphenicol. With antibiotics in hand, we joined the public health doctors and nurses hanging IVs, and the tide was turned. Catastrophe averted.

As it turned out, we were to receive an unexpected reward from the village for our efforts—a weekly basket of mangoes, papayas, and guavas. Thanks, Mactan; sorry Magellan.

In a second memorable incident, there was the bout of mosquito-borne elephantiasis in Leyte. Leyte—where General MacArthur returned in 1944 and where his rusted landing craft are or is still on the beach—had significant public health issues, including malaria and elephantiasis, both mosquito-borne.

One night, after the usual day-long medical field clinic, having seen locals with chronic malaria and several with limbs affected by elephantiasis, my wife, Cande, and I were put up in one of the village nipa huts, a simple but cozy palm-thatched building raised on stilts.

The trouble started at dusk with the room abuzz with mosquitos and no netting to be had. Fearing elephantiasis, fearing swollen limbs, fearing my testicles ending up in a peach basket, we needed to take preventative action. Aside from swatting all we could by hand, we came to a definitive solution. Using the sheets and a bedspread, we created a linen cocoon over the bed where we sought refuge. Lying there belly to belly in the heat and humidity of a tropical night, we realized two consequences—one good, one bad.

The good was that our linen cocoon worked. It was mosquito free. Elephantiasis anxiety averted. The bad—it was sweltering inside, a tropical sauna, a Turkish hammam, a Navaho sweat lodge. So much for charitable public health work. So much for island hopping with public health. So much for wanting to be Albert Schweitzer. Maybe being a plastic surgeon in Beverly Hills would be easier.

Back at the leprosarium, where I was to spend 80 percent of my time involved in the care of severely affected, crippled leprosy patients, I was gaining experience that would unexpectedly turn my interest toward pathology. Specifically, there was one person who had that influence—Dr. Chapman Binford, the chief medical officer (CMO).

The leprosarium had been built in 1928 with funds given by an American, Eversley Childs, in response to an outcome of the Spanish American War in the early 1900s. At the time of the war, several hundred US soldiers were marooned and denied entry back into the US because they had contracted leprosy.

That exile, that requirement for physical isolation in a leprosarium, although emotionally wrenching, was medically rational. Before the era of antibiotics, infection by *Mycobacterium leprae*, akin to *M. tuberculosis*, was contagious. Specifically, military history taught that soldiers coming from foreign battlefields could carry the infectious contagion back home to an immune-naive population. History taught that crusaders returning from the Holy Land in the tenth through twelfth centuries systematically brought leprosy to Europe, with major consequences.

Before the contagion was well understood, it affected tens of thousands throughout Europe as a progressive epidemic until the principle of isolation in a leprosarium was understood. The magnitude of that public health problem can be gauged by the remarkable fact that, at the height of the epidemic during the Middle Ages, there were more than 10,000 leprosaria in Europe. As with most foreign wars (Spanish American, Vietnam, Iraq, Afghanistan), such health effects linger on for decades at great human cost.

In the Philippines in 1921, the newly appointed US governor general was Leonard Wood, who had previously served as both a field commander and a physician in the Spanish American War in the Philippines a decade earlier. Years later, he witnessed the fate of his former now-exiled soldiers, who were to live there in confinement under difficult circumstances for the rest of their lives. Wood worked to remedy the situation by seeking donated funds to build better care facilities.

The most generous donor who empathized with the fate of leprosy patients was Eversley Childs, a New York City industrialist and philanthropist. Under the auspice of the Leonard Wood Memorial Foundation, Childs funded the building of a spacious, well-appointed facility in Cebu. He sought first to ensure care and comfort for the fallen, and second to create a state-of-the-art research facility to ensure ever-improving care.

When I arrived in 1970, some forty years on, the Eversley Childs Leprosarium—still endowed by the Leonard Wood Memorial—was continuing to support patient care and research in microbiology, immunology, chemotherapy, and epidemiology. There was at that time an emphasis on new treatment strategies. All these functions were under the direction of Dr. Chapman Binford, the medical director of the Leonard Wood Memorial Foundation. Binford, a well-known American pathologist, was a distinguished expert in tropical diseases at the US Armed Forces Institute of Pathology. Working with Filipino colleagues, Binford was there to ensure the latest and greatest medical service would be brought to the patients.

I remember being puzzled at the time that a pathologist would be named CMO. After all, weren't pathologists just post-mortem, after-the-fact guys explaining what just happened, not themselves driving what happened?

But that was not Binford. He was the expert who had authored the tropical medicine textbook we all read. His focus was not on the post-mortem, but rather on the here and now, on the mechanism of disease, on the nature of the beast. He had a team of able Filipino MDs caring for the patients. His part was to add deeper understanding. While he was always around, chatting with the patients and other

MDs, he was also leading a laboratory effort to a deeper understanding of leprosy with the intent to improve treatment.

I learned from him that summer of 1970 that the deforming, crippling effect of the disease went beyond the presence of the M leprae bacterium; it was also a profound immunologic response with consequent associated tissue damage. It was akin to scarlet fever and rheumatic fever, with subsequent heart and kidney disease following resolution of the infection. To fully treat the ravages of leprosy meant understanding and addressing this add-on complication that required more than antibiotics.

In the regal presence of Binford, I saw the engagement from patient to lab. I saw his ability to go beyond everyday care to articulate a path to improved care. He made me appreciate the importance of the laboratory-based physician. Whereas the frontline MD touches the patient directly, the laboratory-based physician developing new tests and new insights may touch many thousands—or even millions—as Ventana was later to do. That summer, as a junior neophyte medical student, an unanticipated but important seed was planted. As often happens early in life, it is someone before you who shows you a way not previously imagined.

When I recollected the tales of fighting leprosy, typhoid, and elephantiasis, Mom seemed puzzled. Her memory was fuzzy. She asked what year that was. When I told her it was 1970, she recalled that in 1970 she and Dad were living in Liberia, Africa, on an assignment that lasted from 1967 to 1972. As she thought more about it, she asked, "Was that the year your dad was in Addis Ababa, and they fired a tank shell at the US embassy during a coup? Or was it when he was gone for two months in that camel caravan to Timbuktu to deal with the Gaddafi incursions? Or was it the year he was arrested in Kinshasa in the Congo for taking pictures of the presidential grounds? Or was it the time he was helicoptered into Mogadishu?"

At ninety, her memory wasn't perfect. After all, there was a lot to remember of times past and faraway places. On the other hand, maybe the threat of leprosy or typhoid or elephantiasis in the distant Philippines paled next to her husband being shot at in Ethiopia and Somalia, or dodging terrorists in Timbuktu or fending off inmates in a Congolese jail. On that basis, her selective memory was understandable.

In a family with an extensive library of perils, my exploits ranked second that day.

Mom's recollection of those dangerous events brought us both back to the times when we as a family lived in dangerous places, in dangerous times, back to how it all began, back to Mom and Dad's story.

4.

The Outfit

MOM, NÉE JEAN MACDOUGAL, WAS born in Amesbury, Massachusetts, in 1925. She was the first in her working family of carpenters to go to college. During World War II, in 1942, she made it into the Boston City Hospital nursing program on a path to becoming an RN. But her training was tragically cut short when her mother died in childbirth delivering her fifth child.

With her father off in a combat zone in Italy as a US Navy Seabee, Jean was called home to care for her four siblings. With the help of her aunts, she returned and took charge. She was, after all, of the generation of women whose responsibility to tend to family always took precedence over higher education. She willingly and happily fulfilled her duty, but she never returned to college. This left her with an unrequited need to learn more.

In 1944, she married Dad, Tom Grogan, who was on a two-week leave as a Navy radioman serving on a destroyer on convoy protection from German submarines between New Jersey and Venezuela. They married as he was about to transfer to the Pacific, headed for Iwo Jima and Okinawa. Their marriage came as no surprise to their friends and schoolmates, who had voted them "Most Romantic Couple" in their senior class. I was born nine months to the day after the wedding, and my brother Buzz followed twenty-one months later. Mom was back to home care.

After the war, Dad happily returned to our hometown of Amesbury, a bucolic New England town of 10,000, forty miles north of Boston. Nestled on the picturesque banks of the Powow and Merrimack rivers, Amesbury was home and muse to the famed poet John Greenleaf Whittier. Dad went to work at the family-owned newspaper, the *Amesbury Daily*. But in 1948, he received an unwanted phone call from his former Navy lieutenant requesting Dad return to service. Dad gave him a quick rejection. He'd had all he wanted of war, and the lieutenant knew why. The two of them—Dad and the lieutenant—were the only two survivors in their twelve-man squad. They were radiomen on the USS *Bennington* working with Navajo code talkers who helped them relay secret combat messages to the Marines landing on the beach during the battle of Okinawa.

At the height of the battle, Dad and the lieutenant were headed to the vessel's bridge to deliver a message when a kamikaze hit the *Bennington*. All ten of their teammates were incinerated. That combat left wounds, and Dad preferred to do his healing back home at the printing press rather than on another tour of duty.

Though the lieutenant knew and understood the impediment, he persisted, even going so far as to take the train to Amesbury to plead his case. He explained a new and different kind of war was just beginning—a cold war that was based on information rather than physical conflict. He explained that a Russian spy suspected of working out of the United Nations in New York City was actively engaged in espionage, and the lieutenant's mission was to intercept the coded radio transmissions. The suspicion was that these transmissions were going from NYC to Newfoundland, and he needed radiomen listening 24/7 along the likely transmission route.

The lieutenant stirred Dad's patriotism. As a result, Dad was recruited into the US Navy reserve, but with an unusual stipulation— he was to work only at home, where he was given a large radio receiver. Within a matter of weeks, Dad intercepted one of the first documented Russian espionage transmissions in US history. As a pattern of transmission was discerned and data accumulated, the evidence was taken to Washington. It proved to be one of several threads of information that gave rise to the CIA.

And, as it turned out, the lieutenant was soon to become a key officer in the newly formed communications/cryptanalysis group at the CIA. Within a year, he brought Dad to Washington, DC, and a thirty-year career in communications and codebreaking was born.

Years later, when I asked Dad how they knew it was a Russian transmission, he said it was easy. It was the era of amateur ham radio operators, and the messages were in plain Morse code, mainly in the form of friendly chit-chat. Then suddenly came a message that began with, "*The carrots are on the back burner . . .*" It was an amateurish but definite coded nonsensical message, likely from a spy.

In 1950, the first critical mission of the CIA communication/ codebreaking unit commenced and we—meaning not only Dad, but Mom and my brother Buzz and I—were part of it. All of us were off to the island of Cyprus to live in Nicosia, so Dad and his group could work out of the Royal Air Force (RAF) base on communication intercepts from the U2 spy plane overflights of Russia. And so began our hidden life. We were now part of a secret world, working for what my parents always called "the outfit."

The danger, to begin with, was distant and remote, far away in Russia, but it was soon to get dangerous much closer to home. By 1953, there was a growing revolutionary uprising by the native Cypriots against British colonial rule. That year, the uprising began with a series of bombings of public buildings, police stations, and radio stations. The effort to remove the British colonial yoke was led by an organization known as EOKA (*Ethniki Organosis Kyprion Agoniston*). EOKA called their effort "the struggle for freedom," known by the Greek acronym ENOSIS.

This movement, which started haltingly, escalated as talks with the British failed. By 1954, the violence surged. Assassinations became frequent. Unarmed civilians were executed wantonly in coffee houses, churches, and hospitals. Cyprus in general, and Nicosia in particular, became hotbeds of terrorism. It took an armed British force of 12,000 to contain the violence.

Finally came an EOKA pamphlet announcing, "We have nothing else to do but to shed blood, and this will be the blood of English and Americans," according to Lawrence Durrell in *Bitter Lemons of Cyprus*. These pamphlets, handed out on the streets of Nicosia, set a tone of imminent danger. As our family lived "on the economy" in a Nicosia neighborhood without armed protection, you could say that for the next three years our lives fit the description of living in a dangerous place in dangerous times, with dangerous adversaries.

After the pamphlet, street graffiti called for ENOSIS and promised, "We will shed blood." These very words were once painted on the window of our British Mayflower car, and they've been etched in my memory ever since. We were spending the weekend in the Kyrenia Mountains with our Cypriot neighbor Chris and his family. After enjoying a feast of Cypriot dishes (*mezes*), including *avgolemono* soup, lamb meatballs known as *keftedes*, and honey-baked *loukoumades*, we left the house to encounter a surprise. Our car was painted with graffiti, spelling out the words *ENOSIS* and *WE WILL SHED BLOOD*. I was quickly ushered back into the house while Dad and Chris washed off the paint. On the drive home, Dad addressed the threat, assuring us that families with children were safe. "Not to worry," he said. "Just be vigilant." I remember wondering, *If we're safe, why must we be vigilant?*

I now know, years later, after reading Laurence Durrell's book *Bitter Lemons*,[4] written about this troubled era in Cypriot history, that the British and Americans who made friends with their Cypriot neighbors were in a protected category untouched by assassins. I believe on that day Chris reassured Dad on that point.

As it turned out, we stayed on amid the surrounding violence for another three years. But we were not to remain untouched as promised.

The attack came in December of 1954. Mom was driving Buzz and me to a rehearsal for the church Christmas pageant, and as we turned the corner in Metaxas square, we encountered an angry mob headed to burn the British library. On sight of our British Mayflower, they surged toward us like a swarm of killer bees. As they surrounded us, Mom yelled, "Hit the floor!" as she hit the accelerator. I remember some heavy thumps and radical swerves before she jumped the curb and went off the road through the nearby park. My brother and I stayed down until, fifteen minutes later, we arrived at the church on time for rehearsal. Mom opened the door, pulled us from the car, brushed us off and said sternly, "Don't forget your lines."

As dramatic as these events were, they were not discussed further. The silence, the absence of self-doubt, and the lack of anxiety were all part of getting by in dangerous times. While we were untroubled at the time, this day clearly remained in my subconscious.

In 1963, when I was a freshman at the University of Virginia, I wrote an essay entitled, "I Think My Mother May Have Killed Someone and the Government Had Something to Do with It." In medical school, my best friend—now a Freudian analyst in NYC—upon hearing the story, did some fact-checking with Mom and came back amazed at what he heard. Her explanation for her actions and subsequent silence was that she simply did what she needed to do to protect her children. Full stop. The quick thinking and assertive action she taught us would always be our modus operandi.

When we returned to the States in 1957, we lived in Northern Virginia and settled into an easier life. Dad worked at CIA headquarters at Langley, and we achieved tranquility, meaning Dad was not being shot at, and there were no more riotous mobs. Then, in 1963, I enrolled in the University of Virginia, where I began my higher education.

One unusual aspect of my schooling at both the university and medical school was a stipulation from Mom. My parents would pay for every penny of those eight years. No loans. No debt. But my mom's one requirement was that I never sell my books. I was to bring them home for her to read. And so we commenced an eight-year journey in which she read every book from every class. I remember how annoyed I was to be home on holiday and have her want to discuss the previous semester's books. At the dinner table, she would not so subtly say things like, "So how about Civil War Reconstruction?" Or, during medical school, "How about that new OB/GYN procedure?" Somehow, no matter how circumstances conspired against it, Mom, the congenital intellectual, found a way to glean an advanced education after all.

Years later, after Dad's retirement from the foreign service, Mom was employed as a part-time small-town librarian in Newton, New Hampshire. As a librarian, she rarely loaned a book she had not read, or at least scanned. And, as a grandmother, her birthday and Christmas gifts to all of us were usually books—but not just any books. The books Mom chose for her family were always stories she had first read and loved herself. In retrospect, it is no wonder I grew up bookish with a scholarly bent and ultimately became a university professor.

As for Dad, he led two lives. In fact, he had two identities—one of which was unknown even to his family until his death.

By outward appearances, Dad was an easygoing guy. Engaging and likeable, he seemed to be the average Joe. Having grown up playing hockey in Amesbury, he had an athletic build and the rugged good looks of Sean Penn. His easy demeanor allowed him to blend into the community as a common, everyday family man whose derring-do was never brandished, and whose remarkable feats were well hidden and unnoticed.

At home, Dad was always in motion and almost always good natured and jocular. He was quick to get us out of the house and on to our favorite adventures of hiking, camping, canoeing, sailing, and fishing. Together we camped in the Troodos Mountains and sailed the Mediterranean in our little three-man boat out of Kyrenia Harbour, Cyprus. And he was always buoyant with pride in his sailing crew—made up of my brother and me.

Back in New England, Dad was always ready to hit the woods, searching for a bramble-strewn brook with beaver-built pools. He was always ready to cast a dry fly to a rising brook trout. On those days, the talk was of dry fly patterns like the pale morning dun or the rat-faced MacDougal (a name that always annoyed Mom). If the drys were not working, our talk moved to trico emergers, gold-ribbed hares' ears, and egg-sucking leeches. He was not content to just catch a trout on a store-bought fly. He preferred his own flies tied at the riverside with the hatch in sight. But that was Dad—he always found pleasure in doing and building. Even our cabin on the lake was built by hand one summer by Dad, Mom, Buzz, and me. Working with his hands alongside his wife and sons was Dad's idea of a family vacation. Cabin-building and fly fishing were his antidotes to his other life. Very Thoreau-like and nature-bound.

In startling contrast, Dad's work drew him into an unseen world of cryptoanalysis and clandestine operations. Sometimes he was nearby, at the "listening post" on the RAF base near Nicosia—and sometimes he was off to the souks of Cairo, the casbahs of Damascus, the coffeehouses of Tehran, or the hammams of Istanbul. It might have been to meet with a Mossad man in Tel Aviv or an agent in Amman. His spy craft was practiced out of our sight. It was a covert world of coded messages, letter drops, button-sized cameras, and encrypted code books.

That world was so well hidden that we didn't know until his death sixty years later that Dad had a second government-fabricated identity, complete with a second diplomatic passport. When he was eighty-six years old and near death, an old colleague visited him at hospice and revealed his second identity. The day before Dad died, this friend told me, "Your father helicoptered into Somalia and Mogadishu with me three times, but not as Tom Grogan—as his second identity, Raymond Twiggs." This secret identity came with the territory. Even on his deathbed, his hidden life was shrouded to the loved ones gathered around him, much as it was for Kim Philby. Such is the life of a spy.

Despite the shroud of mystery, one thing remains clear in my memory. In all furtive matters, Dad carried himself with an air of nonchalance befitting his occupation. It was the same quiet confidence that defined James Bond, but this was the stuff of home, not of Hollywood.

At age sixteen, I was told of our family's role in the outfit. I was told only in the broadest terms, of course, and I was shielded from specific details like the existence of Raymond Twiggs. It was always to be the "dance of the seven veils," never more than one or two layers revealed.

Still, as a teenager, learning some of the truth about Dad for the first time, I felt pride and admiration for his derring-do and even his nonchalance. His ease in risky situations was instinctive and unshakable, and risk-taking was organically embedded in our daily lives. His daring was part of our family's foundation, a building block that helped to shape the people we would become. He taught us to focus on the danger before us, not the fright. He taught us that danger was to be met with caution but never with fear, that every problem has a solution, that failure is not an option, and that the answer always lies in action.

5.

An Old Nemesis

AT THE END OF THE summer of 1970, I returned to my senior year of medical school, leaving leprosy and elephantiasis behind me—or so I thought. There was one lingering provocation. It stemmed from a word Binford used that summer that stuck with me, and which I could not shed. It was a word that loomed large in my conscience and in our family history for fifteen years—*thalidomide*. This was the name of a notoriously bad-acting drug that was a powerful sedative and turned out to be a teratogenic disaster in pregnant women, resulting in their babies' loss of limbs (phocomelia) and other deformities. This devastatingly crippling drug had been banned in the mid-1950s by the FDA.

The shock in that summer of 1970 was Binford's mention of the drug. He knew it was banned, but he also knew that it was subsequently proven to be a very effective immunosuppressive, anti-inflammatory drug. And so he placed it on his list of hypothetically beneficial drugs to treat and tame the "immunologic wolves" at play in progressive leprosy. For him, it was only hypothetical and too risky to pursue. He was considering it only because of the dire situation in patients with the immunologic flare-ups of progressive leprosy. He was desperate to eliminate the debilitating neuritis, iritis, and orchitis, the raging fevers and painful nodular rashes of erythema nodosum leprosum. He knew that these symptoms signaled a downward path to patient demise.

Even so, the mere mention of thalidomide by Binford had a haunting effect on me. Fifteen years earlier, my younger brother, Tim—as a consequence of Mom receiving thalidomide to prevent miscarriage in pregnancy—was born with a profound birth defect— an encephalocoele (a congenital ballooning of the lining of the brain) with hydrocephalus, which left him profoundly deformed and mentally disabled.

Tim was born in Cyprus in 1955 and given only days to live. But in a remarkable medical intervention by our family doctor and Mom's obstetrician, and with the help of the US embassy in Nicosia, Tim was airlifted to the hospital at the American University in Beirut, where a Lebanese neurosurgeon performed lifesaving corrective surgery.

That thalidomide-caused cataclysm was to profoundly affect our family for the next sixty years, myself included. For a ten-year-old boy, these were earth-shattering events. I recall all the scary talk of the encephalocoele, the brain damage, the likelihood of peril to Tim and to our family. But the scary was soon followed by the heroic. My parents jumped into action, fighting impossible odds. And the physicians jumped into action too, from the obstetrician who delivered Tim and kept him alive, to the family doctor who attended Mom at home in her bed, to the life-saving neurosurgeon. These physicians overcame the odds. They were of vital, lifesaving importance to Tim and our family.

In retrospect, it was at age ten in these dramatic days of 1955 that medicine became my quest. With the strong influence of their life-saving actions, I wanted to be that life-saving person. And so it was that more than a decade later, in my letter of application to medical school, I recounted those transfixing events of 1955 and expressed my deeply felt need to become a medical doctor.

I remember eavesdropping some months later, on a late-night conversation between Mom and Dad sitting together at the kitchen table. They were discussing thalidomide as the root of the problem. I sensed the anguish their circumstances had brought them and the regret that they were not properly informed. There was an abiding sense of guilt, particularly because the drug was banned back in the US but not in Cyprus. It was a painful, irretrievable liability of living in a far-off place.

It was part and parcel of living in a dangerous place in dangerous times without the customary standard of medical care and protection back home. Today, when I hear public pronouncements thanking military personnel for their service, I think of my parents' less-known service—defending their country against dangerous adversaries—and I think of the unrecognized price they paid for the rest of their lives.

After all the dramatic events, Tim amazingly recovered, and at last we had him with us. This called for a major adjustment, as we now had a fragile baby to care for. Characteristically, there was never a whimper or complaint from Mom and Dad. They were still on mission and on task both at home and at work. Family life was now more demanding and less comfortable, but managing discomfort with unabashed enthusiasm was their well-established, proven occupational strength. In a family where obstacles were always taken as opportunities, we carried on as usual.

As for my personal journey, it was the vivid events of 1955 that directed me to medicine. But in the summer of 1970, fifteen years later, it was our old nemesis, thalidomide, that directed me more precisely to the study of laboratory medicine and the study of the mechanism of disease in the field of pathology, which is devoted to the study of disease.

Fixated as I was, I returned to Washington, DC, and plunged head-on into a deeper study of the powerful immunosuppressive effects of the drug. I wrote my senior thesis on "The Pharmacodynamic Effects of Thalidomide on the Treatment of Progressive Leprosy." It was a twenty-five-page tour-de-force calling forth everything known about thalidomide and pushing further to suggest future applications. It took months to research and write, but it garnered an A+ from a tough reviewing professor. More importantly, that paper was the harbinger of an academic career, as there would later be some 250 scientific papers and a professorship.

That first paper, driven by a "burr in the saddle" that was the ever-lurking thalidomide, hinted at a future academic life. I had found my scholarly doppelganger. I had found what Thoreau called my inner "vital heat."

It is funny how a single word among 600,000 in the English language can drive one to a higher purpose. But drive it did.

While Binford and that summer inclined me to the study of tropical diseases and pathology, global events in 1971 took over, leaving leprosy, thalidomide, and elephantiasis behind. Namely, the war in Vietnam was in its ever-expansive mode. By June of 1971, when I graduated from George Washington Medical School in Washington, DC, on the heels of the Tet Offensive, every graduate of a US medical school was drafted for military service. And soon, in July 1971, I ended up at the Letterman Army Medical Center in San Francisco for a year of internship in internal medicine.

Internship is when you're molded into a physician through total involvement and commitment to the patients before you. It's medicine 24/7. You are all in, day and night. Internship is when the dough is kneaded and becomes a loaf. It is when clay is turned into a pot. It is when letters become words and words become sentences. It is when you achieve medical literacy through total immersion.

Thoughts of leprosy behind me, I settled into hospital rotations in cardiology, gastroenterology, pulmonology, hematology, oncology, and the intensive care unit. The goal was to master hands-on medical care.

Oddly enough, absorbed as I was in the everyday care of patients and finding great satisfaction and a sense of purpose in it, I was to be drawn once again back to pathology based on a specific experience—my interaction with the head diagnostic pathologist at Letterman, Dr. Bill Doyle.

My interaction with Doyle, the all-knowing, egg-headed diagnostician, was prompted by an ongoing circumstance. In every ward that year, typically with thirty to forty patients under care, there were always three or four patients who were a mystery, who defied clear diagnosis. It frequently was the biopsy read by Doyle that gave us certainty. As the intern responsible for many of those difficult patients, I often found myself at the two-headed microscope, knee-to-knee with Doyle, being shown the definitive answer. It was the eagle-eyed pathologist like Doyle who knew what was going on inside a patient, and thus was often the one who led us to the proper diagnosis and treatment. From Doyle, I learned the diagnostic pathologist was not the post-mortem, after-the-fact guy. Rather, he was sometimes the only-one-who-knew guy. I wanted to be that guy. Right then and there I signed up for a residency in pathology at Letterman.

Since achieving national certification in pathology meant acquiring encyclopedic knowledge of both anatomic and laboratory medicine, I was to spend the next four years in residency, from 1972 to 1976, at Letterman.

Over those four years, I was schooled daily by two masters—the ever-present Doyle and the ever-influential Dr. Gist Farr. As time went by, Dr. Farr was to have an increasingly pivotal effect. He was a bespectacled, owlish Southern gentleman, born wise, who came from Memorial Sloan Kettering Hospital in New York City, where he had trained with two of the living icons of pathology, Drs. Frank Foote and Fred Stewart. As we all were during Vietnam, Farr was fulfilling his military obligation, in his case in a teaching capacity. And teach he did, fully armed with encyclopedic knowledge of pathology gained from Foote and Stewart. Under Dr. Farr's tutelage I had the daily experience of being held to their high standards. Dr. Farr was the mentor who taught me the path to excellence and to mastery. Since Foote, Stewart and Farr were experts in cancer diagnosis, I acquired a like interest.

Besides the requirement for encyclopedic knowledge, there was another profound influence by the Foote, Stewart, Farr school— mindset. They saw the diagnostic pathologist as an active primary director of care, not a passive participant. They fully articulated the critical role of the up-front diagnostician known as the surgical pathologist. This was the pathologist right in the middle of the surgical suite, doing frozen sections and directly influencing surgical care. After all, proper surgical care requires not only knowing the extent but also the nature of the disease.

There was one more seminal influence during my residency. That was a two-week elective I spent in surgical pathology at Stanford, just twenty miles down the road. There I was to witness pathology at the next level, an even more aggressive practice of surgical pathology. At Stanford, the diagnostic pathologist was stationed right by the surgical suite in what was called the "hot seat." From that perch, the pathologist was in and out of the operating room, handling the surgical biopsies, cutting and staining the tissue on the spot, and calling the diagnostic shots. It was the pathologist as quarterback. And having played quarterback in high school, it fit my personality. I liked calling the plays.

This aggressive directive form of surgical pathology practiced at Stanford was organized by professors Richard Kempson, MD, and Ronald Dorfman, MD, who came from Washington University in St. Louis where they had trained under another icon, Lauren Ackerman, MD, who was the author of the surgical pathology textbook we all used in the 1970s. Ackerman was the main proponent of the highly active, assertive school of surgical pathology. I had found my people, and my aspiration then was to train further at Stanford.

Compounding my aspiration was my experience at Stanford of witnessing the latest advances in chemotherapy and radiotherapy for cancer, particularly malignant lymphoma. It was the dawn of the era of newly formulated "combination" chemotherapies and the great excitement of realizing the first cures. I saw world-class laboratory science applied to guide therapy. I saw the Binford model used in lymphoma and I felt I had found my exact calling—to become a hematopathologist. It's funny how two weeks can set you on a course of forty years. But once you have set your course, left the shore, and gone to sea, the currents can be too strong to turn back.

The exciting part was that I had found my goal. The tricky part was that I still had two more years of obligatory military service. At the time, getting into a fellowship at Stanford seemed impossible.

That uncertainty aside, based on having received high marks in training, I was given a plum assignment as head of the hematology laboratory at Walter Reed Army Hospital in Washington, DC. That was the reward for past accomplishments. There was soon the thrill of being at a famous 1,200-bed, tertiary-care hospital with 120 beds dedicated to hematology. Walter Reed presented every unusual, strange, and perplexing medical case on the planet. It was to provide me a lifetime of experience in just two years. That was the thrill, but there was also the fright. There were always ten to twelve perplexing patients outside the realm of textbook knowledge. As a rookie on my own, every night was a late night.

Compounding the stress was the fact that Walter Reed was the hospital for the US Congress and the White House, so many cases were of high visibility. Imagine fielding a call from a senator on the Ways and Means Committee regarding his wife's diagnosis of lymphoma. I was a rookie playing in his first World Series. To gain assurance and to ensure diagnostic authority, I needed outside help. That outside help came in abundance when I asked a distinguished hematopathologist, Cos Berard, at the nearby National Cancer Institute to assist. Bringing Cos my difficult biopsies on a weekly basis, I quickly found my guru. As busy and famous as he was, he always gave me—and my difficult patients—his time. As he later confessed, his inclination to help came from the fact that twenty years before he had the same job I did and understood the need for assistance.

As the year passed, both our common history and weekly involvement with patients bound us together. One day, nine months on, Dr. Berard said he had a surprise for me. As we sat at the microscope, he picked up the phone and called his close friend and colleague, Ron Dorfman, the professor at Stanford. Right then and there, he suggested to Dorfman that I was an ideal candidate for a fellowship at Stanford. It was a bit of a staged event—knowing of my aspiration to go to Stanford, he had previously called Dorfman. He just wanted to see the joy that came over me in the moment. And joy there was. There is no greater elixir than a mentor who believes in you and promotes you to others.

Based on that strong recommendation from Dr. Berard, I was to start a fellowship in hematopathology at Stanford the next year under the tutelage of Dorfman, Henry Kaplan, and Roger Warnke. It was there, from July 1978 to July 1979, that I experienced my third career-transforming event. There in Warnke's laboratory I was introduced to and schooled in the newly born field of immunohistochemistry (IHC). It was in the Warnke lab that I learned the methods of by-hand tissue biopsy chemistry. I learned that probes (antibodies to proteins, oligo nucleotides to DNA and RNA) tagged with dyes (red, brown, and blue) could paint invisible cells and thereby make them visible under a microscope. My eureka moment was the realization that the entire repertoire of proteins and nucleic acids (DNA, RNA) could be demonstrated and studied using a standard light microscope. The entire inner universe of more than 200,000 proteins and 30,000 genes could now be visualized in every cell, in every biopsy, in every patient. By these methods, I learned there was an immense inner universe that could now be explored, that could now be used to explain the inner workings of cells and also to detail the molecular derangement that could explain the mechanism of disease and suggest new targets of therapy. Suddenly, I had in hand the new tools to think like Binford.

The fact that each test was very labor intensive and time consuming was not an intellectual barrier but a physical one.

Solving that problem through automation lay in the future. In the meantime, with new tools in hand and a few publications to boot, I was able to land an academic position at the University of Arizona Medical Center in Tucson in 1979.

In retrospect, all things considered, it was the seed planted by Binford, nourished by Doyle and Farr, watered by Berard, and fertilized by Warnke and Dorfman that was to grow into a seedling at Stanford. The seedling, then transplanted in Arizona, matured and came to fruition in my pivotal year of 1984.

As I recounted my intellectual journey, a smile came to Mom's face. She reminded me that it wasn't all work, and that in my third year of residency at Letterman, I had squeezed in a six-month course in French pastry, working through the entire French baking repertoire. She reminded me that I had learned to make Jacque Pépin's *dacquoise aux* chocolate, Gaston Lenôtre's *gateau marjolaine*, the almond-paste pithivier, and Dad's favorite, *babas au rhum*.

My talk of training in San Francisco and Palo Alto came back to her oddly as a vivid gastronomic remembrance. Her remembrance was understandable, since in the years after Dad retired in 1974, they often came out to sunny California from snowy New Hampshire. They came to associate their visits with these new and exotic tastes.

It's funny how a ninety-year-old manages to retain a precise sensory memory, while other memories slip. That night, her strong culinary flashbacks trumped talk of medical training and other details.

Her memory was rosy, and I didn't trouble her with the backstory. I had never told her—and wasn't about to tell her—of my act of truancy. She never heard that I used to slip out of the hospital on Thursday mornings for those six months to go to cooking class. My truancy was made possible by my fellow chief resident, Jim Fitzwater, who covered my tracks in exchange for a weekly pastry sample.

In retrospect, my truancy could have gotten me sent to the front lines in Vietnam. My truancy was the kind of thing that happened in the days of a drafted army but is quite unlikely in today's professional Army.

Anyway, I didn't want to trouble my ninety-year-old mom with my deceit. Rather, we reveled in her gastric glee.

6.

Blue Sky

CATHERINE'S CALL TO "BUILD SOMETHING that can" was a call to invent. The need was for a new tool, an instrument that *could* provide physicians with more accurate, expedient diagnoses for their cancer patients, as well as provide the volume of tests the hospitals needed.

Besides Catherine and I, the Grogan Lab at the University of Arizona at the time included graduate PhD students, MDs in training, and scientific fellows. These would-be inventors were cell biologists, immunologists, biochemists, medical scientists, and medical students—not an engineer in the lot. Inventing and then building a never-before conceived instrument would require professional engineers, and to use it in medical practice would require professionals from the medical device industry. We had none of these, but we were unconstrained.

Like the Wright brothers 120 years ago, running a bicycle shop in Akron, Ohio, imagining motorized flight, we were not engineers, but we were too keen to invent to let it go. And like Leonardo sketching a helicopter 500 years ago, long before electric motors, we were too full of imagination to let practicality—or reality—stop us. As any young couple with a child will tell you, conception is too easy and too much fun to be outsourced. Raising the child is another matter altogether.

The laboratory environment, with its mix of technicians, graduate students, medical students, and fellows, was soon to contribute strongly to our urge to invent. In particular, the graduate students became a major creative force. Give a graduate student an arduous, demanding, repetitive, boring job, and they quickly become creative geniuses. While they loved the excitement of biologic discovery with each new antibody, they loathed the drudgery of doing the chemistry by hand. The reagent preparation, the bucket brigade of solutions, the need to work under a hood with masks and gowns, and the constant clang of a timer calling them to the handling of the glass slide, all added up to a numbing, laborious day-long intrusion on their intellects. According to Adam Smith in his 1776 *Wealth of Nations*, the factory system, with its arduous repetitious work, turned workmen into inventors. In 1986, 200 years later, Adam would find his "repetition fuels imagination" theory upheld by handwork-averse graduate students.

The measure of this inventive Adam Smith equation began to occur precisely every Friday afternoon, when we held our research meeting to review the week's findings and to plan for the next week. To begin with, the topic of automation was a fifteen-minute sidelight, a bit of mental gymnastics, for the fun of it. It was just talk, but soon it morphed into more. It morphed into concepts scribbled on the blackboard, into sketches in lab notebooks. The students' minds were soon doing what their hands didn't want to do. Their thoughts were beginning to take physical form. Conception was upon us all.

They began to meander and tinker endlessly, and we eventually came to what the chairman of the pathology department, Jack Layton, called our *blue sky* phase. You might expect this unplanned, unfunded, preoccupying phase would be upsetting to a chairman who had recruited me from Stanford, had given me lab space, funds for technicians, and 50 percent of my time free from hospital duties. He had invested a lot. Surely, by the usual academic expectations, there would now follow a proper academic progression: generation of research data, published papers followed by government grants, and funds to repay the department. We were eventually to do all these things over time, with more than 250 scientific papers and more than twenty-five years of grant funding. But that was to occur years later.

Jack was not the typical chairman. He set a different expectation. Six months after I arrived at the University of Arizona, the lab was established, Catherine was hired, and I was to report our progress to Jack. We had publishable results, and we would now proceed to seeking grants. The surprise was his answer.

"I'm pleased with your progress," Jack began, "but I recommend a mid-course correction."

"A course correction?"

"Let's hold off on the grant applications for now."

"But isn't that how I am supposed to repay the department?"

"Yes, in due time. But for now, hold off on seeking grants. It will only get you bogged down in the time-consuming chase for minor iterative advances wanted by some distant committee of scientists. Why not take the time to do something more original, more daring? I think we both have time for that. Let's go for more than the usual. Let's go for a little *blue sky.*"

At the time, I wasn't quite sure what Jack meant by "blue sky," but I understood perfectly well what I had just been granted: time, space, resources, and political cover. I now had a mentor, a protector, and an expectation to invent. I was given the freedom and the funds to go unconstrained. I was free to meander and not be committee driven. I was free to tinker. I was free to "escape necessity," as prescribed by Seneca, the Roman philosopher. Advising independence, Jack had freed me from what he called copycat grant work. I was set adrift, to be carried away on ocean currents to *terra incognita*. I felt like Darwin in 1830 on the *Beagle*, headed for the Galapagos.

After months of weekly lab meetings, I finally sat down one day with a yellow legal pad and sketched a few drawings, giving physical form to our ideas (see Fig. 3). These doodles translated all the talk and ideas into visible form. The drawing took the world of 1 x 3-inch

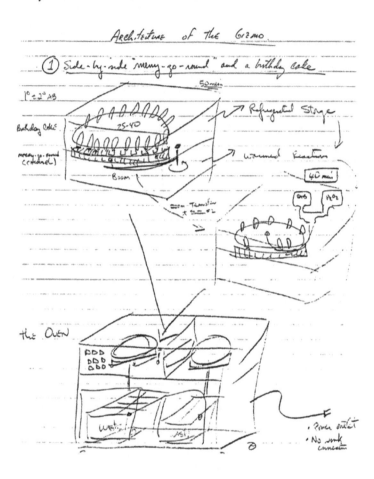

Fig. 3. My original 1985 drawings labelled "the architecture of the gizmo." This was one of a series of six sketches I used to translate all the talk and ideas into physical form. It took the scattered world of 1 x 3-inch glass slides and the bucket brigade of chemical solutions (reagents) and envisioned a refrigerator-sized instrument to house all the key elements. It containerized reagents in dispensers (what looks like candles on birthday cake) and moved the glass slides from reagent station to station on a carousel that has remained a key feature on our instrument for over thirty years.

glass slides and the bucket brigade of chemical solutions (reagents) and envisioned an instrument that housed all the key elements. It containerized reagents in dispensers, and it imagined at least one dynamic element, an actuator or plunger to automatically dispense reagents. This eliminated the human labor associated with hand pipetting. As amateur inventors, we were pleased at our envisioning of this mechanical advantage.

Later, when real professional engineers were involved, this simple mechanical gain was seen as horse farmers being pleased with a new-found "mechanical horse" instead of a tractor. Even so, this first amateur conception articulated some pivotal architecture that remained relevant for thirty years and through three generations of instruments. There were two other substantial benefits to those drawings.

I now had images to show and persuade others—images to suggest a business possibility—and I had images that would be used later in an important patent filing. Mom wanted to see them.

"Let's leave the lab and the hospital," she said. "Tell me again the story of how the company began."

With visions of a medicine-changing instrument in mind, my thoughts shifted from dreams and doodles to reality. How might I actually build an instrument, now affectionately known from the drawings as the *gizmo*? Clearly, I would need professional engineers and chemists, and to get them I would need money. And to change not only our lab but labs everywhere, I would need big money, say tens of millions of dollars. To get it, I would need venture capital, but first I would need to recruit real businesspeople with knowledge of the medical device industry and then generate a business plan, and to do all that, I would have to be a legitimate business. Alternatively, I could have outsourced everything or sold the idea to others, but I was too far in to do that.

Before I could contemplate starting a business, and before I could recruit others to our cause, I had to face one major constraint—I had been branded a Class 6 felon.

Being a felon eliminates any prospect of gaining funding or recruiting anyone except perhaps other felons. Being a felon was also decidedly incompatible with the term "legitimate" business.

Armed as I was with a well-conceptualized, inventive idea, likely very useful to doctors and their patients, who could have imagined being branded a felon? But branded I was, by the lead attorney, T. Thompson, at the University of Arizona, after I sent him a copy of my recently obtained Arizona business license enclosed in a letter seeking permission to proceed with a formal business.

I was seeking permission because as a faculty member of the University of Arizona medical school, I was a state employee, and— by state law—I was forbidden to form a private business while on the public payroll. In fact, as Thompson explained, I was likely already a Class 6 felon based on my filing for an Arizona State business license. Evidently, the fifty dollars I paid for the license was about to cost me a whole lot more, with future employment now in question.

The legal ruling was definitive and unequivocal; permission denied, reality found. As I struggled to accept this legal reality, I contemplated an alternative. Perhaps I could negotiate with Thompson for part time. Coming from Stanford, why not suggest what Hewlett and Packard did in the 1950s as graduate students in electrical engineering. They bargained for a day away each week to pursue their idea in exchange for Stanford receiving shares or equity in their enterprise. Permission given, Stanford received considerable Hewlett Packard (HP) stock and great economic gain. In retrospect, the HP, or the *Bill and David equation* of equity for permission, and the subsequent success of HP, taught us all that universities could create economic gain by connecting and licensing to industry. This way of thinking fueled the technological boom in the Bay Area known today as Silicon Valley.

With these thoughts in mind, I called Thompson to try to find the middle ground.

"I understand state law says no company," I began, "but how about permission to dabble part time, say an afternoon a week, as Hewlett and Packard once did?"

Thompson was unmoved. "No dabbling, no funny business. Tear up the business license, eat the fifty bucks, and all is forgiven."

"Well, how about the example of HP and Stanford and all the good that came from that?"

"Stanford is a private university and thereby free to make the rules as they wish. We are a land-grant state university. We're publicly funded, you are a state employee, and you are therefore subject to state law. Nice try! Now tear up the license and let's call it a day."

Knowing the legal ruling was definitive, knowing my suggestion of an alternative swapping time for equity was out of the question, unequivocal defeat was at hand. Knowing when to hold 'em and when to fold 'em, I folded. It was time to return to the academic monastery. I had jumped the garden wall, was caught, and now I needed to confess and show contrition. It was, after all, better to be contrite than a felon. And so back at the monastery, a few days after I folded, Jack Layton, my department head, came calling.

"Have you heard from the university attorney?" he asked, knowing full well that I had.

"Yep. It's a definite NO, an unequivocal NO. Absolutely against state law. I am to cease and desist and tear up the license, or I am a Class 6 felon."

"So, what have you decided?"

"I'm folding. I'll tear it up and let it go."

"Just like that?"

"Yes, because my parents didn't send me to medical school to become a felon."

It was at this low point that the unexpected occurred. As I slumped and retreated, Jack went the other way. In a flash, he was on his toes like a rooster about to crow. And crow he did!

"Alright then," he said. "There is only one way out of this. We will have to change state law. I believe the university will gain by giving licenses to its faculty in exchange for equity. That's it. We will change state law to allow a conflict of interest in exchange for full disclosure and the university gaining equity. I know just the guys to help us, but first you must not quit."

"Yes, sir."

As I sat stunned in his office, struck by the impossibility of Jack's plan, he swung into action. He was on the phone, and the next thing I knew I was sitting across from the dean of the College of Engineering, Dean Dahlin, who took me down the hall to the office of the university president, Henry Koeffler. He was to take the proposal to the Arizona Board of Regents, who called in the head of the legislature, Burton Barr, who wrote up and pushed through a new state law known as Arizona House Bill 4284, wherein a public university employee could engage in private enterprise, if disclosed and if the university was granted equity.

From start to finish, the whole process took months, but suddenly I was out of jail and now considered a shining star of daring and innovation, an icon of the new economy. But for all the subsequent publicity and hoopla, the reality was far more mundane. After all that effort, all I really had was *permission*. I had a license to hunt but no weapon. Big deal. Now came the hard part—raising money and recruiting colleagues. We probably needed a hundred million dollars and a few dozen well-paid professionals willing to take a risky, lower-paying job in a company likely to fail.

But for the moment, all future difficulties ignored, gaining permission was an important positive milestone—a testament to our resolve. It was also a testament to the importance of alliance. My daring, able, risk-defying allies included my chairman Jack Layton, the dean of engineering, Dean Dahlin, Koeffler, the Arizona Board of Regents, and the head of the Arizona legislature, Burton

Barr. What they all had in common was a belief that academia and industry would both benefit from drawing closer. Koeffler saw this as the University of Arizona rightfully acting on its mandate as a land-grant university to improve the economic well-being of the great state of Arizona. That, after all, is what Lincoln had in mind in the 1862 when he signed into law the land-grant bequest.

Most remarkably, Barr, the head of the legislature, took this enthusiasm to another level. He drove a rare bipartisan approval, espousing intellectual property and enterprise coming out of the university as a new form of real estate, albeit *intellectual* real estate. And if there was one thing members of the Arizona legislature understood and coveted, it was a land grab. In the long term, Burton Barr was to be proven right that universities, including state universities, could drive the state economy by spurring private enterprise, which promotes manufacturing and employment.

Mom, having met Jack, reminded me that he was a quintessential Iowa farmer, and ran the department like a farm: the hens will lay, the cows will be milked, the pigs slopped, the corn planted, the wheat harvested. Running Jack's farm involved the whole family, and at the end of the day they were all to sit down and eat together. Once a week we were to attend the faculty meeting as if going to church— not to be skipped without risk of your immortal soul.

Jack understood that the eggs, the milk, the bacon, the corn and the wheat had to be harvested, brought to market and sold for a profit to keep the farm running. This experience fueled his belief and support of me engaging in enterprise. He saw academics as another type of farm, sowing ideas, producing new tools of value and creating economic gain in the marketplace. Jack was an intellectual farmer.

With permission brewing, it was time to focus on raising money and recruiting talent outside the lab. Having no money and no ability to pay anyone for anything, I began recruiting others with the only thing I had—the quest. This had worked already in the lab, but now we needed a real businessperson to join the quest.

Oddly enough, that process began on the basketball court. Not just any basketball court, but in my neighbor Darryl Dobras's backyard where we played one-on-one basketball. Mano a mano was our sport. We both liked the elbow-to-elbow, in-your-face, give-it-all-you've-got to twenty-one points competition. It was the physical antidote to our work week, my time in the hospital and his at his architectural firm, restoring historic buildings.

Between games, sitting on the court in sweats, I invariably started talking about the lab and the gizmo. You know how a friend keeps on a repetitive theme, and it's going nowhere but they can't let go? Well, eventually that's what it came to. This was the exchange.

"You are a typical academic." Darryl was annoyed. "You can talk endlessly about an abstract topic. You can even make drawings. You might even write and publish about it. But for all the yammering, you will never actually build it. Enough already! I'll find you a real business partner, but you need to stop talking and get going on it. Now let's get back to playing."

And so I was spurred to further action. But more importantly, Darryl, as a man of action—true to his Viking heritage as a marauding Norseman—was then to help in two important ways. First, true to his word, he connected me with and helped persuade an experienced businessman, Ross Humphreys, to join the quest. Second, he was to add his voice to the process at the university in his capacity as board member of the University of Arizona Foundation.

Darryl gave that very important assistance expecting nothing in return. In later months, when Ventana came into financial success and I offered him compensation, he'd always decline, citing his prior family experience. He explained that when I spoke of inventions and instruments, of intellectual property and a startup company, it reminded him of his own inventive father-in-law back in Lorain, Ohio, who as an engineer had founded a startup based on his electronic inventions. Darryl had witnessed the benefits to his hometown and family through employment and economic gain. This remembrance spurred his own philanthropic motivation. He had seen it before and he was determined to see it again, with no compensation required.

Darryl persuaded Ross, who also joined the quest without pay. He was a graduate of the Wharton School of Business, returning to Tucson after working for McKinsey Consulting. He had returned to Arizona with his wife from a pioneer Arizona family to live on the family's homesteaded land, with an eye to start his own enterprise. Ross was to give us a sound, well-articulated, well-organized business foundation. He wrote the first business plan, and he joined in the negotiation for university permission to proceed. He organized our effort to raise money. He brought in local capital from Jim Strickland at Coronado Venture Capital (CVC). He recruited the first employees after raising the first money and organized pursuit of the big money. He became our first CEO and was the backbone of the operation. Ross set the standard for hard work, total commitment, and total daring.

He used his Wharton and McKinsey connections to get us venture capital interviews, but it was rough going. We were two guys out-of-pocket with limited means, some drawings and a made-up business plan. We were easy to dismiss.

Our first success came from an interview with the head of business development at a Bay Area medical device company, Becton Dickinson (BD). They gave us $50,000 to conduct a marketing survey. Specifically, we were to document three customer feedback sessions (focus groups) with practicing pathologists to test the likely adoption of our idea. We were to document what is known as the voice of the customer (VOC). Working with a marketing firm, we found ourselves behind a one-way mirror observing the discussion of our idea with local pathologists in New York City, Philadelphia, and Chicago.

The first two sessions, New York City and Philadelphia, were disastrous. In both instances, the consensus was rejection. Both groups said they already had what they needed. Their diagnoses were accurate and a device to add chemistry findings would be an unnecessary expense. They could not imagine a future delivering a report on the mechanism of disease. It didn't seem possible, so why waste time working on the unimaginable? About the best the Philadelphia group could do was to imagine a faster hematoxylin and eosin (H&E) stain—the primary diagnostic stain in use for more than one hundred years. That reaction brought to mind what Henry Ford said regarding the lack of imagination of a horse-drawn population before his automobile. Ford said, "If I asked a guy on a horse if he would like an automobile, he would have said, 'No, I prefer a faster horse.'" Like Henry Ford, our survey of customer needs was underwhelming.

Even so, with our remaining $15,000, we flew to Chicago—where it all went the other way. There we found a group of young, imaginative, energetic pathologists who were so enthusiastic they called for a chalkboard and commenced to break into working groups and design their own instrument. We had what we needed—someone, somewhere who thought we were right! Actually anyone, anywhere would have been just fine.

Back in the Bay Area, sharing the tapes with the BD crowd, they agreed, having been shown the Chicago tape first. Then, when brought down by seeing the other two tapes, I filled the gap by saying New York City and Philadelphia were the unimaginative VOC; Chicago was the imaginative VOC, which we referred to as the Voice of the Cognoscente. Quite a stretch, but they bought it and decided to proceed with a promise of funding several hundred thousand dollars.

As it turned out, we never got that payment, and we also ended up returning the $50,000 with $10,000 in interest. That's because Ross had successfully interested a small local Tucson venture fund (CVC), which came in with several hundred thousand dollars, on the condition we return the $50,000 to BD to ensure there was only one thumb in the pie. That venture capitalist, Jim Strickland, gave us the means to hire our first recruits. As often happens with venture capitalists, he gave us more than money; he gave us his time, his expertise and his wisdom. He was a positive factor in recruiting our first engineer, Chuck Hassen, our first biochemist, Jim Rybiski, and our first medical device scientist, Phil Miller. These three gave us the engineering, chemistry, and medical device savvy that led to making our first prototype, known as a *breadboard.*

Thanks to Jim, we also rented a small garage-like space in a strip mall with an open office and a few engineering benches. Thus was founded our *Navy 6 SEAL* unit, with Ross Humphreys, Jim Strickland, Chuck Hassen, Jim Rybski, Phil Miller, and myself. We soon had a prototype instrument based on more professional drawings, and new chemistry formulations. We had money in the bank and a genuine payroll. It was time to go for the big money, and to go for filings for intellectual property (IP), including patents and trademarks. We proceeded with boundless optimism, unaware of the pain to come.

Looking back, I still marvel at how we were able to recruit jewels like Chuck, Jim, and Phil.

Chuck had a degree in mechanical engineering from MIT and a business degree from Harvard. When he moved from MIT/Harvard to the edge of the intellectual universe, Chuck went from being just another brilliant person in Boston to one of the smartest guys in Tucson. His creative engineering brought the gizmo to the next level. Many of our foundational patents came from Chuck.

Phil had twenty-plus years of experience in inventing and developing medical device systems at Abbott Labs. Phil knew how to marry the hardware and the chemistry to make a hospital-worthy instrument. He knew how to proceed to build a new system. He was a born inventor, and he too gave us many pivotal innovations.

Chuck and Phil both had far more secure positions with far less risk and better compensation than we offered. Why risk it? Because, as I learned from them and many others we were to recruit over the years, the quest mattered. The idea of a new field— of new inventions, of instruments and tests never built before, of transforming medicine—was magnetic. So, we always put the quest front and center.

As for compensation, there was not comparable pay, but the carrot was stock options. At the time, Ross had set up the structure, and our Ventana Medical Systems, Inc. (VMSI) stock was valued at 63 cents a share (even though we all knew that price was arbitrary and most certainly ridiculously overvalued). For all the uncertainty of value back then, the stock was worth nearly $90 a share twenty-two years later when our company was acquired.

Beyond the appeal of the quest and the stock options, there was also the joyful enthusiasm factor of "come work here and have a lot of fun." We called it "the Tom Sawyer factor," recalling the incident in Mark Twain's *Adventures of Tom Sawyer* in which Tom is stuck white-washing Aunt Polly's fence when his buddies come by to go for a swim. Spotting them from a distance, Tom starts whistling joyfully and whooping it up. His buddies are soon drawn in to share the joy and fun by grabbing a brush and joining in the work detail. And so, Ross and I did a lot of joyful whistling, and exuded a lot of enthusiasm and optimism, and handed out a lot of paintbrushes.

7.

Big Bucks

TO PROCEED FROM CONCEPT TO development—from R to D—required capital. Not millions of dollars, but tens of millions. And so with drawings, a few slides to project, and a thirty-minute presentation, Ross and I headed to the temples of venture capital in Silicon Valley, Chicago, Dallas, and New York City. In an eighteen-month span, we presented to thirty-five venture capital sites and received thirty-five rejections—about two a month. The rejections, though unwanted, were professional and polite. Typical rejections went something like this:

This is a naive proposal from an unwitting academic.

We don't think it's the kind of business an academic should be dabbling in.

You will not be around for the tough part. You're all R and no D.

Those were the ad hominems. There were also the non-personal rejections of the idea that went something like this:

This kind of esoteric technology would never make it out of university.

It's a long-term project taking five to ten years to profitability . . . yet we have computer deals that give three to five times return on investment in two to three years.

This is a slow boat to China, not the speedboat we seek.

We only invest in the big returns of pharma and therapeutics, not the small margins of diagnostics.

We have run the idea by several groups of practicing physicians, and they don't see the need.

Your method of chemistry on a glass slide, to interpret a biopsy with a microscope, to make a subjective qualitative judgment is trumped by flow cytometry and PCR methods, which are quantitative, analytic, and objective.

Imagine proposing marriage thirty-five times, with thirty-five rejections. It was probably time to go to into the priesthood with vows of chastity or—in my case—to return to the monastery, to the academic sanctuary of medical school, seek forgiveness, and give up whoring with capitalism.

Then something unexpected happened. A righteous twig snapped. As tough as they were to take individually, none of the rejections were substantive. They were amply skeptical, but they were also unwitting of the workplace, unwitting of the part of medical practice that needed to change. They were unaware of the often-unspoken uncertainty of diagnosis. The physicians they solicited were not forthcoming about their foibles. The venture capitalist investors were also unaware of how adding chemistry (IHC) to every biopsy would be transformative. The venture capitalists didn't know what I knew. I resolved, righteously, not to quit until I got a true, have-all-the-facts, definitive, scientific, medical rejection.

And so I slogged on, awaiting that final definitive dismissal. Seeking that ultimate rejection, I changed my approach. I pared the thirty-minute presentation down to twelve minutes. It became the well-honed elevator speech. It was just the facts, take it or leave it, yes or no, no obliquity.

Our thirty-first rejection came after fifteen months of effort. It was consistent with prior rejections, except this one—unlike the others—was abrupt and impolite.

The rejection came on home turf. Venture capitalist Phil Brown flew in from Boston to see the lab, the drawings, and the breadboard, and to hear the pitch. This was the second visit. The first, by his partner, Jim Weersing, was enthusiastic. In a pattern I now knew well, the first visit was the good guy—the cockeyed optimist—and the second was the bad guy—the back-to-earth skeptic.

I understood the odds. Before me was Mr. No Go, but the first was so enthusiastic and our pitch so well-honed that our optimism was alive and well. And so, after a brief walkthrough meeting and greeting the lab techs and fellows, we ducked into the conference room for the now-polished twelve-minute elevator speech, the pitch of pitches. Curtain up, lights on, show time! This was to be the Academy Award-winning performance.

Then came the shock. Two minutes in, Phil sat shaking his head. Not a little, but a demonstrative, repetitive, horizontal head-wagging rejection. I stopped my pitch.

"Excuse me. We're just two minutes in and I'm already being rejected? Really?"

He responded, "Forgive me, I am being quite rude, very impolite. I'm very sorry, but please understand, I flew in last night on the red-eye from Boston and I am a bit frazzled." And then came the killer comment—the unequivocal, unanswerable dismissal.

"I know I should be more polite, but it's not just the lost sleep. Your idea, your invention is also the problem." I begged an explanation. He obliged. "You see, the company we just started in Boston has a Nobel Laureate as a founder, and he is taking us into the scientific stratosphere. And your idea, well, it's not rocket science. It is far more practical, let's say very earthbound. Sorry."

There it was, an abrupt, impolite, unanswerable dismissal. To be seen as mundane, humdrum, lacking in imagination, and earth-bound was the lowest of the low. This was the intellectual *coup de grace.*

At this logical quitting point, this moment of defeat, came a surprise. Suddenly, out of the lull, came the last flaming ember of mental reserve. Without hesitation—as I had learned from the thirty previous rejections that hesitation itself was lethal because it demonstrated a lack of mental agility—I shot back. My rebuttal to the unanswerable went something like this:

"I hear you. You're right; this is not rocket science. It is not Nobel-worthy. It is merely practical. But the category of Nobel versus practical brings to mind Maxwell and his brilliant conceptualization and mathematical formulation of the propagation of light, a truly Nobel-worthy abstract intellectual feat. As opposed to Thomas Edison, whose more practical idea on the propagation of light was to impede electricity with a carboniferous filament in a vacuum to produce incandescence. For all its mundane practicality, Edison's light in a bulb had the virtue of allowing one to stay up at night, after work, and read about Nobel-worthy work like Maxwell's mathematical equations. Given the everyday universal utility and economic value of Edison's light bulb, I would have thought you as a venture capitalist would bet on Edison over Maxwell."

Phil smiled. He was suddenly polite. He had found the spark he was looking for. He began to speak in sweeter tones. The call from Boston two days later showed a hint of true interest—it was a tentative maybe. At last, at least a *maybe.* The exhilaration of a less-than-total rejection.

As it turned out, a few months later success came with presentation number thirty-six—and soon thereafter, Phil Brown and Jim Weersing joined the enterprise as the number-two investor, and both were to stay with us for the next twenty years, until the acquisition. And so, all facts considered, it may be said that in the end, thanks to Thomas Edison, the practical prevailed over the abstract.

After eighteen months, thirty-four rejections, and one maybe, success came at last with presentation number thirty-six. The audience was just one person, John Patience (JP), who saw what the other thirty-five did not. JP was a venture capitalist at a small Chicago venture firm. It was JP who first realized the opportunity and seized the moment. Like all the rest, he was skeptical at first. After all, I was just a medical academic with a few drawings. But unlike the others, who saw only risk and a long lead time to return on investment, JP saw the medical promise. He did something no one else had—he came to the lab, sat at the scope, and witnessed the ongoing drama of the hospital. He was drawn to the medical detail of patients being diagnosed and treated. In particular, JP's interest lay in the patients whose diagnoses I had changed, and where their care had been altered. He wanted to hear more.

Answering his request to hear about the *"changed"* patients, I presented four patients with a couple of PowerPoint presentations, each taking about three minutes. There was the thirty-eight-year-old mother of four with misdiagnosed and mistreated breast cancer. There was the eleven-year-old with highly treatable Hodgkin's lymphoma, misdiagnosed as carcinoma and mistreated to deafness with the wrong drug—cis-platin. There was the fourteen-year-old in a coma who was misdiagnosed with meningitis, but who had a lymphoma. Finally, there was the ten-year old boy falsely diagnosed as having a lymphoma in the tonsil who had infectious mononucleosis.

I had presented these same cases to the other venture capitalists in PowerPoint form, but JP was simply more inquisitive. He was drawn to the medical detail. Unlike all the others, he asked to come to the lab to hear and see more. Unlike the rest, he wanted to see the biopsies, and see the chemistry, to understand the reasons for the misdiagnoses, and to learn how our invention was able to ensure correct diagnosis. Having broken the twelve-minute elevator pitch mold, we sat down at the microscope to discuss the details and see the findings in the scope, spending a full hour on just the first case.

First, the clinical detail. Our thirty-eight-year-old mother of four, Mrs. Smith, with misdiagnosed breast cancer was mistakenly thought to have an estrogen receptor–positive invasive ductal carcinoma. This led to her receiving, post-surgery, anti-ER therapy with Tamoxifen. She was assured that her cancer was ER-hormone dependent, and therefore denying it estrogen on top of the surgery should prove curative.

The error, the misdiagnosis, was the estrogen receptor finding. The ER positivity had been determined by the laboratory standard-of-care test at the time, by the biochemical assay for ER, which was quantitative and precise with a standard error of 2 percent. This was the national standard assay, "precision medicine" at its best, because of its analytic accuracy and reproducibility. It satisfied all the rigorous requirements of laboratory science.

Despite its analytic accuracy, it happened to be the wrong finding in this patient for a precise reason—the assay was performed on breast biopsy tissue that was ground up in what is called a *grind-and-bind* assay. This grinding of the tissue mixed together both the cancer and the normal glandular cells. It was not until two years later, when the breast cancer recurred as a metastasis to her liver, that we discovered the error. The surprise was that the liver metastasis of breast carcinoma was ER-negative. How could that be, given the primary tumor was ER-positive?

At Mrs. Smith's request, we returned to study her original biopsy. That was possible as only half the tissue had been grind-and-bind; the other half was fixed and embedded in paraffin. When we sectioned that original block, keeping the whole biopsy intact with cancer cells and normal cells in their respective places, the true biology was revealed.

At the microscope, looking at the chemistry on the glass slide, JP saw as I did that the ER signal was in the normal breast cells, and not in the adjacent cancer cells (see Fig. 4). As it turned out, she never had ER-positive ductal breast cancer. She was ER-negative and should have been treated differently, with chemotherapy. At that moment, JP understood what we were doing, what it meant to see the chemistry of the cells in context, what it meant to have a probe (the anti-ER antibody) with chromogen (dye) paint the intact cells to see microscopically what was otherwise invisible. This is what it's like to know the true nature of the disease.

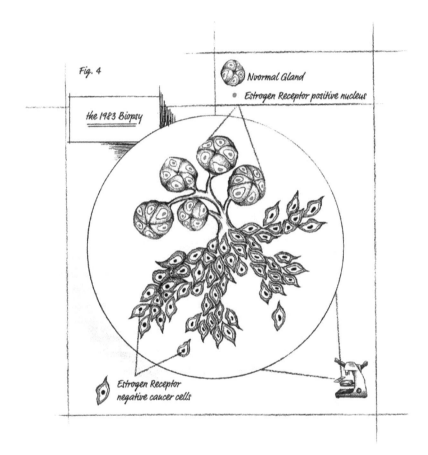

Fig. 4. Mrs. Smith's biopsy, showing an invasive breast carcinoma mistakenly called estrogen receptor positive. This illustrates the reason for the mistake. The estrogen receptor (red) is found in the normal, round, regular breast gland cells, and not in the irregular invasive cancer cells (absence of red). The mistake was made by the test-tube biochemical method, which began with grinding up this tissue (bind-and-grind methodology), so there is no distinction between normal and cancer cells. Our tissue immunohistochemical (IHC) method kept the tissue intact and allowed the distinction between normal and cancer cells.

JP, as an analytic, linear thinker, understood from this case that the quantitative, objective grind-and-bind assay was analytically precise but medically and biologically imprecise. It failed to distinguish between normal-ER and cancer-ER expression. He quickly understood that the holistic IHC method that kept the tissue intact allowed a more precise diagnosis. He understood that MDs do not simply treat lab results, they treat patients. He understood that a diagnostic pathologist using a microscope, seeing the whole picture, adds medical judgment to the chemistry to achieve certainty. From this, JP—unlike the thirty-five others who preceded him—understood the need for change, the need for new tools, new chemistry and new automation.

As for the risky-business fear of all of the others, JP saw it differently. Not naively, not unquestioningly, just differently. He knew that our business plan, predicting financial success within three years, was naive. He knew my request for a few million dollars would not cut it. He knew it would take more like $150 million to $200 million to produce a medical device worthy of FDA approval and a global business. He knew it would take eight to ten years.

To JP, these financial obstacles were surmountable. It was not the financial risk that prevailed in his thinking. He was focused on the patient side and the need to improve and transform medicine. His own wife's agonizing fight with cancer, her suffering, magnified his awareness of medicine's inadequacy in the false promise of cure.

And so it came to pass that JP was all in, both analytically and emotionally. He brought us his financial, intellectual genius. He gave us the business foundation we desperately needed. He soon thereafter brought in Jack Schuler, former CEO of Abbott Labs, to start a two-man venture fund, Crabtree Ventures. Schuler was to give us his bedrock medical device business experience, which was also critical.

JP and Jack, committed as they were to transforming medicine, were always seen by Mom as truly worthy members of the assembly of like souls. As I retold their tale one night, they joined us around Mom's bed.

With the big bucks in hand, we had to do what we promised, and every penny would be needed. There was no luxury in the equation. We were not passengers on the *QEII* eating caviar and sipping champagne, destined for the Riviera. We were more like crewmembers in the engine room of a tramp steamer eating hardtack, headed to Terra Del Fuego. Luxury, no; shoveling coal, yes.

We used our new funds modestly, as every startup knows it must. Our first priorities were to hire more people and increase our space. The six of us, crammed into a small garage-like office, had successfully produced a prototype instrument worthy of the big money, but now it was time to go to a production model and develop chemistry to match. To these ends, we quadrupled our space by renting offices in a strip mall. To call them offices was a euphemism; it was actually four cavernous garages with tiny broom-closet offices. The idea was that the cavernous space would allow us to build a makeshift laboratory, and we thought the clever part was that the spaces could all be interconnected.

After we moved in and furnished the place with makeshift laboratory benches and used furniture, we discovered some not-so-clever parts. Namely, we were unwittingly located half a mile northeast of the city sewage treatment plant and we were just thirty yards from the major transcontinental Southern Pacific Railroad tracks, which we learned moved trains hourly with a noticeable clamor. Add in a welding shop next door, and you had all the trappings of a true startup, modesty attained.

As it turned out, our overzealous commitment to modesty had a significant impact on our objective to recruit others. Imagine trying to entice a university-bred PhD or engineer from Boston or Connecticut to a strip-mall garage near the railroad tracks at the edge of the known universe. Those challenging interviews went something like this:

If the wind was blowing from the southwest, our out-of-town interviewee, upon exiting the car to enter the "plant," would come under olfactory assault. There was an unmistakable smell of a barnyard, of a pig farm, of a feeding lot. It was a smell of rotten eggs and ammonia of planetary proportions, as in the atmosphere of Venus. The interviewee, now aghast, looked at the interviewer (often me) as if I had just come in from slopping pigs, or escaped from a nearby cholera ward. Once we were inside and sitting for the interview, the offensive odor typically diminished, but with occasional bursts of rotten eggs and ammonia. Needless to say, the interviewee under olfactory assault didn't take the job, concluding, *This place stinks. I am not leaving Boston or Connecticut for this. I would rather sack groceries at Safeway.*

And so it was, we were done in by prevailing westerlies, done in by a force of nature. Startups fail for many reasons, but to fail because of the wind blowing from the southwest would be unique in the annals of startup failures.

Every problem begs a solution, and mine was as follows: Early in the morning, I would check the weather section of the *Arizona Daily Star*, and if the wind was brisk from the southwest, I would conduct the interview at a hotel. On meteorologically favorable days, I would confidently conduct ammonia-free interviews onsite and generally did so with great success, provided I accounted for one more factor—the Southern Pacific Railroad schedule. Compared to the more stinging ammonia, the railroad effect was more discreet, though sometimes disquieting.

The railroad effect went something like this: The interviewee and interviewer seated at chair and desk, in a fully oxygenated room, free of ammonia, would at first experience a slight tremor. It began as a mild vibration moving to a more persistent vibration, often jiggling objects on the desk. The interviewer would at first pretend to rearrange papers on the desktop, but as the vibration turned to a teeth-rattling rumble, all pretense vanished. The interviewee would go into alarm mode, wondering if the train was about to roll through the room.

This sense of impending doom dampened any serious scientific or business discussion. The interviewee, though smelling nothing adverse, left the premises concluding that it was not smart to seek employment at a place that induced a sense of doom on an hourly basis.

We, of course, learned quickly how to overcome the doomsday effect by consulting the Southern Pacific Railroad schedule and avoiding in-office interviews at key times.

And so on meteorologically favorable days and at favorable railroad hours, we were able to focus on the exciting work ahead and enjoyed great recruitment success. That was, until the ant colony took over the building and started biting, but that's another story.

Anyway, on days that didn't stink, didn't rumble, and didn't bite, we signed a few high-draft choices.

8.

Kodak Moment

WITH THE BIG MONEY IN hand and recruiting in process, the focus moved from a makeshift breadboard prototype to a full-on production model. As soon as Chuck Hassen and Phil Miller recruited their high-draft choices, they left amateurism and cartoons behind and professionalism was afoot. While they saw some virtue in the cartoons regarding architecture and mechanics, they saw them for what they were—sketches of a mechanical horse imagined by horse farmers. After thoughtful analysis, both drew the same conclusion: *Forget the mechanical horse. What we need is a tractor.*

To make a tractor, to deliver a transformative system, they were to go beyond the mechanical functions to the command-and-control functions, the dynamic kinetic functions that would not just replace human labor but also drive speed and save time.

By using microprocessors and lasers, new to medicine in 1988, they gained machine-driven control. By adding pneumatics (compressed air), they drove mechanical functions like the mixing of reagents on the glass microscope slide, which sped up assay times. By employing LCD screens and codified microprocessor recipes driven by laser beam–scanned barcodes on the glass slides, the operator was in total control. After adding the barcode label to the slide to specify the test desired, the operator could simply push the button and walk away. This was automation, ahead of its time, akin to what Eastman Kodak did for the Brownie automatic camera with the slogan, *You push the button, and we'll do the rest.* This was our Kodak moment.

There was one other aspect similar to Kodak's—the pre-packaged, containerized chemistry. As it turned out, our chemistry was to become very similar to Kodak chemistry on a cellulose membrane or film. Kodak's most important invention was not the camera but the film chemistry, and so it was for us. While the added machine features gave us great gain over hand labor, there was considerable invention relevant to our film chemistry, which was new to the field and was itself transformative.

Thanks to Phil, the chemist and system integrator, and his able assistant, Jim Rybski, the chemistry went from a bucket brigade of solutions and a last-minute mixing exercise to a set of snap-on dispensers containing all the prepackaged, barcoded reagents. One particularly important problem solved by Phil and his team was the stabilization, containment, and dispensing of the key color agent or dye known as diamine benzamine (DAB), which was a Class I carcinogen. Ironically, the lab techs were assisting in the diagnosis and cure of cancer by using something that caused cancer. Before Phil, the lab tech had to handle this powdered, volatile, breathable carcinogen DAB by working in a medical-class safety hood with air controllers while wearing gloves, gown, and mask. Imagine that as part of the everyday routine on top of the bucket brigade.

Phil's ability to formulate that DAB, containerize it, and dispense it free of gloves, mask, and gown was a major improvement in workplace labor and safety. In later years, we often sold this attribute to the hospital safety officer and lab manager.

Among the key inventions by Chuck and Phil were several brilliant ideas. The first came by adding command-and-control functions by a microprocessor.

Chuck had brilliantly conceived and orchestrated all the complex and interlevened instrument functions and recipes on his own microprocessor, which via a floppy disk allowed universalization of recipes to all instruments. This universal brain was to become a key to lab automation.

Even so, there remained a critical issue—how the operator was to interact with and command the instrument. How was the microprocessor (computer) to know which of the fifty tests was to be started? How was the computer to know which of the twenty-five steps in fifty different recipes were to be followed? The human interactive element, even if it was just to state intention, was still needed.

That need for human–machine communication remained unsolved until one day when Chuck went grocery shopping. While standing in line watching the barcode-driven, laser-scan checkout of a customer with a basket full of items, Chuck thought that a barcode laser-scan system might work in medicine, too. Forget the price and inventory on macaroni and cheese; how about the recipe for an ER or a HER2 assay?

Grasping his eureka moment, Chuck added a liquid crystal display (LCD) interface to the barcode/laser-scanner system and in one fell swoop gave the instrument more than just a brain—he gave it a means to communicate. Suddenly, Hal (as we called the computer) could communicate with Chuck and others. Now our machine's nervous system not only had a brain, it also had a peripheral sensory system. Thanks to the laser scanner, it could see the barcode on a patient's glass slide that detailed the test parameters. And thanks to the LCD it could communicate to a human. Chuck had found the inventive, transformative combination at the grocery store. And so it is that deep thought and invention are not confined to the workplace; sometimes a grocery store will do.

Whereas Chuck and his teams' inventions resulted from pursuit of better command-and-control, Phil and his team were focused on faster assay results by driving the chemistry. Done by hand, at ambient temperatures, the reactions occurred slowly by simple diffusion. The opportunity with machine control was to gain speed by adding controlled heating. Besides heat to speed up diffusion, there was a second important consideration called the *unstirred layer effect.* This occurs when there is a reaction on a solid glass surface like a microscope slide whereby the reactants line up like a picket fence, slowing down diffusion. The answer to this picket-fence effect was machine mixing (see Fig. 5). By hand, neither heating nor mixing was used in practice for obvious reasons. The first was the difficultly of handling heated glass. The second was the impracticality of hand-mixing each slide.

The combination of machine-controlled heating and mixing accelerated the time to equilibrium of the assays. However, the combination produced a more confounding effect—evaporation. The greater heat and more rigorous mixing drove evaporation, resulting first in a loss of temperature control and second in drying the glass surface, which stopped the assay in its tracks. So, Phil and team, to gain speed and time, had to control three factors: precise heating, uniform mixing, and evaporation.

The first issue, precise heating, was easiest to solve, using microprocessor-controlled thermistors. In contrast, controlled mixing proved more daunting because Phil had made an unusual, tricky choice. He chose to use the microscopic glass slide as the reaction chamber. This might be considered an illogical choice, since the flat-planed glass had no walls. How was it to hold solutions? Wasn't it illogical to have a wall-less chamber, a glass without sides? How would it hold water? The answer was a reliable force of nature— capillary action. This is the strong attraction (surface tension) that

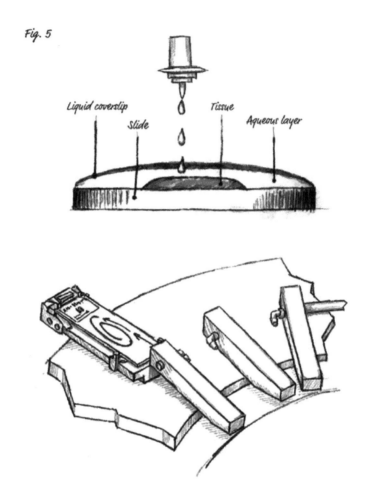

Fig. 5. Key inventive components of the automated instrument (the "tractor").

Top: The wall-less chamber. Pictured is a glass microscope slide (side view) holding a "puddle" of chemical solutions (reagents), held to the edge of the slide by capillary action. As the puddle is heated to drive the reaction, the potential evaporation is contained by a thin layer of oil (the liquid coverslip). As shown, reagents may then be dispensed from above and washed off at will.

Bottom: Shown is the dynamic mixing of the dome-shaped puddle with a well-controlled compressed air jet. By this means, we achieved uniform mixing.

occurs when a liquid interacts with a solid surface. Phil learned that by capillary action, a 1 x 3-inch flat glass microscope slide could hold 100 to 150 microliters of fluid quite effectively without spillage. Thus was born the reaction chamber without walls as shown above.

There were many virtues to the wall-less chamber. Because there was no physical barrier, reagents could be added and removed at will. There was no chamber to clean or remove, no disposable to handle. It allowed hands-off chemistry. Chemistry could be added from above, from dispensers, by gravity. Now some of the time-sensitive reactions, like the addition of hydrogen peroxide to activate DAB to go from colorless to a visible precipitate, could be mixed on the fly. No more last-minute mixing in the hood with mask and gown. This meant the carcinogen DAB could be dispensed, contained, and mixed without human contact. It also meant the reactions could be terminated by simple flooding. This was an open system that allowed an endless variety of combinatorial chemistry on a slide in an individualized barcode-driven manner. Lastly—and most importantly for patient care and safety—each reaction was unique to that patient's individual slide with no reused chamber. Carry-over from patient to patient was therefore not possible, and safety was ensured. The result was individualized and unique to that patient alone, not part of a batch of slides in a common chamber.

Thus was born the idea of a chamberless, open, automated, individualized tissue biopsy chemistry. Here was an instrument doing what a human could not. But for all the virtues of the wall-less chamber, it created a daunting problem related to mixing, which was vital to speed up diffusion. How were we to push around microliter quantities of liquid on a glass surface without walls? All of our attempts to vibrate, jiggle, and jostle the slide failed as the commotion invariably overcame the capillary action and knocked the solution off the slide. After weeks of painful trial and error, the team at last achieved a novel solution— compressed air. It turned out that the dome-shaped puddle on the glass slide was easy to push around with a well-controlled compressed air jet. By this means, the delicate balance between commotion and capillary action was found and uniform mixing achieved.

For all the inventions, for all the benefit of heating and mixing in wall-less chambers of individualized chemistry, there remained yet another daunting, unsolved problem—evaporation. All that heating and mixing with hot air over the puddle greatly enhanced evaporation. The problem of evaporation was compounded by the wall-less chamber. There was no physical barrier to constrain the heat-driven Turkish bath we produced on the slide.

This became the showstopper. This was the problem beyond invention. This was why no one had done it before. No matter how hard you push it, an elephant cannot fly. This time, there were no magical forces on our side. Forget the wall-less chamber, forget blue sky; return to reality, and admit defeat. The frustration of this fatal flaw loomed for agonizing weeks. We were down to hand-wringing and antacids. It seemed like it might be the right time to see if our old jobs were still available.

For all the agonizing and all the effort, the solution was not to come at work. It was not to come from design committee meetings. It was to come from jogging—while seeking physical solace from mental stress—and from seeking total workplace detachment. The solution came to Phil while he was jogging in Sabino Canyon among the ocotillo and the armed saguaro cacti. It's a funny thing about the frontal cortex and cerebration. It sometimes does best when relieved of duty. Sometimes it takes the balm of splendid isolation and discontinuity to fuel original thinking.

On that jog, while pounding the ground, Phil in a flash had his eureka moment. Why not float lighter-than-water oil over the slide-bound puddle? The puddle of fluid would be snugly covered by the evaporation-resistant oil. The only real question was whether the oil would reduce the surface tension holding the puddle. After a hasty return to the lab, PM showed with a few experiments that indeed the oil blocked evaporation, and capillary action held. The wall-less, oiled chamber worked!

As for the instrument, the solution was simple—a discreet squirt of a neutral light oil. Further experiments showed that all the chemistries dispensed from above passed through the oil by gravity without altering activity.

Mission accomplished.

Tragic flaw overcome.

And so the newly invented combination of heating thermistors, compressed air mixers, and anti-evaporation oil ushered in what we called *hands-off, automated, speedy, kinetic-mode immunohistochemistry.* Our moniker then was to be like Kodak. "You push the button, we do the rest."

It was time to turn our gizmo into a medical-practice-worthy, FDA-worthy, hospital-worthy, global-worthy instrument.

To view a video of the instrument in action go to www.tgroganmd.com.

With our key invention in hand, it was time to proceed to a commercial product, but we also had to take the time to document every technical advance and file for patents. In the first iteration, there were more than eighty patents filed. To be patent-worthy, an invention must be a novel idea reduced to practice. For example, evaporative control by a film of light oil was unquestionably new to medical devices, and by our constant use was reduced to practice, so a patent was readily attainable.

Our novelty multiplied by eighty, giving us a unique system protected by a bundle of patents. This patent portfolio was a key asset, as we were later to present ourselves to Wall Street. The protected base of intellectual property was a quintessential necessity for a sustainable capital investment-worthy biotech company.

An interesting sidelight was that the patents were not just in the names of the engineers or PhDs. Also named were technicians, who often contributed to reducing the novel ideas to practice. As I participated in that iterative process, contributing my own ideas, I was named in fifteen of those patents. For several of these, I was named as the *cartoonist,* an oft-used designation in patent law crediting the physical visualization of an idea. It takes all kinds to secure a patent; it takes an intellectual village.

After all the technical talk, Mom asked me to return to the stories of our patients. Like John Patience, she always wanted to hear about the lives we had changed.

And so we stopped talking of instruments and inventions and recalled that in all the drama of the ever-evolving business, I had always kept at practicing medicine and always drew inspiration from my patients.

9.

Tadpoles, Caviar and Muskox

IT WAS 9 A.M. ON May 23, 1992, in London. Twelve of us were happily ensconced in a cozy conference room at the Royal Society of Pathology near Buckingham Palace. It was to be the first meeting of the newly formed International Lymphoma Study Group (ILSG). We were twelve mid-career professors from eight countries out to redefine our field. We would combine our accumulated knowledge gained from making new antibodies, and from doing chemistry on tissue biopsies of a malignancy of lymphocytes known as lymphoma.

One of our revered founding members, Dr. Peter Isaacson, was to start the proceedings by presenting a series of patients with a radical finding. They all had a form of stomach cancer, what he called a mucosa-associated lymphoma, which unexpectedly began not with a genetic change but with a bacterial infection. The infection led to persistent inflammation that over time slipped into malignancy as simply as a tadpole becomes a frog.

As he spoke, an uneasiness grew. It was against all medical dogma, against textbook knowledge. How could an infection lead to cancer? Inflammation and cancer were unequivocally separate. One related to infection, the other to genetic mutation. How could this be?

The infection he described began with a well-known gastric inhabitant known as Helicobacter pylori, or H. pylori. This bacterium had historically been regarded by the medical community as harmless. It was thought to be a friendly member of the gastrointestinal flora, which sounds almost botanical—natural and beneficial. This assumption that the bug was harmless was to be proven incorrect. The infection by H. pylori was subsequently proven in 1982 to drive inflammation and hyperactivity, resulting in a peptic ulcer and bleeding. This finding was established by two Australian physicians, Robin Warren, a Perth pathologist, and Barry Marshall, an internist. Warren, with the mindset of Chapman Binford, made the crucial observation, using silver staining on biopsy sections, that this heretofore unsuspected bacterium was present near peptic ulcers. Warren took it a step further, bravely self-administering H. pylori, leading to his own peptic ulcer. The two subsequently won the Nobel Prize for their work in 2005.

Before this finding was published in 1982, virtually all physicians were skeptical since we were trained in medical school that ulcers were related to personality, not infection. We were taught that ulcers occurred in over-wrought, neurasthenic worrywarts, best controlled and best treated by antacids, protein pump inhibitors, and a stress-free work environment. Putting it on the patient, the suggestion would be for a long vacation in Hawaii or Bora Bora followed by daily meditation. The Australian doctor's self-infected demonstration put an end to the blame game and rightfully shifted treatment to antibiotics and H. pylori eradication.

By the time we met on that fine May day in London, we knew of this link between H. pylori and peptic ulcers and the need for antibiotics. But the surprise was Peter's revelation that the inflammation surrounding the ulcer, over time, if untreated, evolved and turned malignant.

Hearing and seeing the evidence, there was a growing uneasiness in the room, which suddenly felt less cozy. Why the discomfort? Because as the presentation progressed, the implication was clear. We the expert diagnosticians had been the ones over the years delivering these diagnoses, which often lead to radical treatments including surgery, chemotherapy, and radiotherapy. Had we really been misdiagnosing and wrongly treating all these years? We the experts! How could the global experts on malignant lymphoma be so wrong?

It was in this moment of deeper reflection and regret that Peter hit us with the clincher. He began by showing us a gastric biopsy, which we all agreed was malignant lymphoma needing both surgery and chemotherapy. But, as he explained, this patient had received neither. In defiance of conventional wisdom, he instead received triple antibiotic therapy with total resolution of his lymphoma. At this news, there was an audible gasp in the room. Peter had acted on the assumption that antibiotics might work early on, while the cells were still driven to grow by the H. pylori and before permanent genetic change occurred, and this patient upheld his radical assumption. You could get the tadpole before it became a frog.

At the instant of that revelation, I was compelled to flee the room and call home to Arizona. The call went something like this:

"Operator, get me the head of the clinic—Dr. Miller."

"Dr. Grogan, what's up?" Dr. Miller asked. "Calling all the way from London?"

"Regarding the twenty-eight-year-old that I diagnosed last week with gastric lymphoma, scheduled for gastrectomy and chemotherapy . . . do not do it! Give him antibiotics instead!"

Dr. Miller was incredulous. "You want me to cancel surgery and give him antibiotics. What? Are you crazy? His gastric mass is bleeding profusely and if I don't remove it now he may bleed out. And then, if I don't give him chemotherapy, it may spread."

I then related all that I had just learned. Dr. Miller, always a good listener, said, "Alright, how about a reference?"

"There are none."

"Why not?"

"The manuscript is in review."

"I cannot base unconventional therapy on unpublished just-heard results from a clubhouse in England."

I pressed him. "Look, if I am right, the antibiotics will be curative. If not, support him with transfusions and then go to surgery and chemotherapy."

Dr. Miller was getting agitated. "Okay, but if you're wrong and he dies, they will sue us, and so they should, and I will have you on the stand before the jury first, so you damn well better be right about this!"

Then, in an act of daring and trust predicated on our ten years of practicing medicine together, Dr. Miller, who was never a fan of gastrectomy anyway, gave the patient triple antibiotics, and then, slowly but surely, the malignancy, the mass, the ulcer and the bleeding resolved within three weeks—without surgery—to the amazement of all involved. The gastrectomy was avoided, and the twenty-eight-year-old left free of H. pylori and with an intact stomach.

As often happens in our field, the best medicine is characterized by what does not happen: a stomach not removed, an infection not persisting, a peptic ulcer not present, a mass not evolving to genetic mutation, a patient not in a clinic. Looking back, it might seem a triumph; after all, a twenty-eight-year-old's stomach was saved, except for the sad recollection of all the past patients over generations treated more radically before Isaacson, before we understood it was an infection and not an anxiety disorder. In contrast with the best medicine is the worst medicine. In this case a failure to identify the root cause of a pathology, a failure to determine the nature of the beast, a failure to find the mechanism of disease. We thought it was *nervous*, when it was in fact *infectious*!

Another important painful lesson was to be learned over time. For all the excitement and favorable results with this patient, we learned from many more patients that only half of them respond to antibiotics because, for some, the gastric mass evolved to incur genetic mutations, which immortalize the cancer cells. Learning this, early detection before genetic change became an imperative. And so, from that May in 1992 on, thanks to Isaacson, every stomach biopsy was to have either immunohistochemistry (IHC) or the very same special silver stains (SS) used by Robin Warren for H. pylori because the imperative was to find and treat the H. pylori before genetic change. Get the tadpole before it becomes the frog. The governing principle came from Hippocrates's oath to first tend to the care and cure of your patient, which we translated to the imperative, "Miss no cure."

Thirty years on, our tests for H. pylori remain one of Ventana's most-used assays globally. Importantly, the silver stain and its variants allow identification of numerous infectious organisms, from H. pylori to fungi, to pneumocystis carinii in tissue sections. Additional special stains allow identification of mycobacterium tuberculosis and M. leprae.

The criticality of these tests to the practice of medicine led us to develop a separate special stains instrument, now available worldwide. After all, it would now be malpractice to leave an infection untreated with antibiotics and, in the case of H. pylori, to allow it to evolve to lymphoma and to have missed a cure. Hippocrates would certainly agree.

Finally, the H. pylori story teaches us there is a huge potential with IHC and SS to facilitate cancer prevention. Another excellent example, detecting early cervical cancer, is told in a later tale.

Misdiagnosis can change a person's life cruelly and profoundly. I learned this lesson in 1994 at a conference table in France.

It was on April 9 of that year in Toulouse, at our third annual meeting of the ILSG, that I learned of yet another misdiagnosed and mistreated entity—the *undifferentiated malignancy*. It was given this name because it was a rapidly growing, metastatic tumor that appeared primitive under the microscope. The root cause was unknown, hence no rational therapy.

At this meeting, professors David Mason (Oxford), Harold Stein (Berlin), and George Delsol (Toulouse) revealed a newly discovered root cause. Having developed a new probe (CD30) for a rare type of lymphocyte, they found the root cause using IHC. The tumor was a malignancy of the lymphocytes—a lymphoma. And again, because it was so primitive, they called it *anaplastic* (without form), and the new entity was named *anaplastic large-cell lymphoma* (ALCL).

They presented a series of patients previously diagnosed as undifferentiated malignancy but now identified as ALCL. They emphasized that virtually all these patients died untreated, but two treated with radiotherapy survived. They suggested that this frighteningly bad-looking, bad-acting tumor was highly amenable to radiotherapy and chemotherapy. Although they had not published the results yet, their advice was to go home and spread the word.

After returning from Europe, I was to present in Chicago at the semi-annual Southwest Oncology Group (SWOG) meeting in my role as head of the SWOG lymphoma biology committee. And so, standing before more than a thousand oncologists from 225 medical institutes, I presented the findings of this new entity of ALCL. After the presentation, as I was leaving the auditorium, an audience member approached me.

"I think I have what you just described," he said.

"You look perfectly healthy to me," I responded. "Not like someone under lethal threat."

"No," he said, "I don't mean just now. I mean twelve years ago. Back then, in Florida, I was diagnosed with an undifferentiated malignancy in my chest and sent home to die. But, as a medical doctor and a radiologist, I insisted on at least some treatment, so I was given radiotherapy. Within weeks the tumor resolved, but I still returned over the next twelve years for quarterly follow-up exams because I was constantly reminded it was highly likely to recur. I ended up living on cancer probation for the next twelve years. Instead of living every day, I was dying every day. Or so I thought. Given my story, do you think I might have had an anaplastic large-cell lymphoma?"

"Possibly," I replied. "Send me the paraffin tissue block of your biopsy, and I will analyze it for CD30."

This was possible through the generosity of Mason and Stein, who sent all of us home from the Toulouse meeting with a vial of the anti-CD30 antibody. Within the month, our radiologist patient sent me the block, and sure enough, it was a CD30+ ALCL. All of this was done before Mason, Stein, and Delsol published and before commercialization of the antibody. That's the way it was thirty years ago in the pioneering era of IHC.

I sent a written report to the patient in Florida, giving him the diagnosis of ALCL with all the details of the chemistry performed. Within days, there was a phone call. The conversation went something like this:

"Thanks for all you have done, but are you sure?" he asked.

"Yes, I am sure."

"Am I cured?"

"Probably."

"Not good enough," he pressed. "I need a more definitive answer."

"Well, I am just the diagnostician, not your treating physician."

"My treating physician doesn't even know this disease entity exists. I need you to say I'm cured. Look, for the last twelve years I have lived every day as if it was my last. My wife and I have cruised around the world twice on the *Queen Elizabeth II*. We have taken ten supersonic flights on the Concorde. We have visited thirty-four countries and dipped our toes in the waters of every Caribbean island you can name. I have gone sky diving in California eight times, and bungee jumping in New Zealand. We have flown all twelve family members for a week in Paris. I have bought my wife a mink coat and the largest diamond I could find. Every night, we dine on caviar and champagne and molecular cuisine. I cannot keep this up. I'm exhausted. Am I cured or not? Tell me now!"

"Well, for the sake of your future mental health, I am compelled to say you are most definitely cured."

"Thank you! Hallelujah! No more circumnavigations, no more supersonic flights, no more molecular cuisine. Back to burgers and fries and baseball."

"Baseball?"

"Yeah, I was a huge fan but had to give it up because of my cancer."

"Why?"

"I gave it up because I couldn't afford to watch a sport with no definite time limit when my own time was limited."

And so he returned to normalcy. We had not changed his treatment or his treatment outcome, but we had informed him about the true nature of the disease, and for him that deeper understanding had a benefit. It helped him live more assuredly. As he told me after, "The way you live matters. When I look back, I realize I was pretending I was living it up every day, but underneath I felt like I was dying every day, and twelve years is a long time to be dying. Now I feel like just plain living every day. Thanks for shedding more light on my path and giving me better assurance and peace."

As for the medical science that benefited our radiologist patient's sense of well-being, it required crossing the borders of Berlin and London, of Toulouse, of Chicago, and of Arizona in order to help someone in Florida. As we learned from our radiologist, the best medicine is global, and without borders.

Who knew that a musk-ox pot roast would come from being waylaid on the Niukluk? Who knew that being an expert in lymphoma would have anything to do with salmon fishing in Alaska? I didn't.

Standing waist deep, drifting a feathered hook to entice a silver salmon, my thought was more contemplative than inquisitive. Standing alone in the pristine, crystalline Niukluk river, deep in the Alaskan tundra near the Arctic circle, my concern was not for another fish; after all, there were already two back at camp, which had been *ulued* and set on alder to smoke. And the migration up from the Bering Sea was full on, so the silver salmon were coming easy. My thoughts rather drifted to the splendid solitude found on those endless mid-August days. The serenity brought me to recall the refrain of the Alaskan poet Robert Service, who asked of the wilderness wanderer, "Have you strung your soul to the silence?"

I was close to that meditative state, hearing only the trickle of water over pebbles, when the silence was broken by the whine of an engine and the sight of a boat coming right at me. The intrusion, while sudden, was not unusual because in that part of remote Alaska any human encounter calls for a courtesy safety check. Usually, it was just a slowdown, a wave and a thumbs-up. But more than the usual passing wave, this was a full stop and a call for conversation. Goodbye, Robert Service.

I greeted my intruder happily, as he was a well-known guide on the Niukluk. Tom Gray was a half-Inuit, half-Norwegian big-game guide for bear and moose, a salmon guide, a reindeer farmer, and a woodsman par excellence. His presence was welcome but unexpected, as he was not the guide who had dropped me off. That would be Ron Davena and his Inuit wife, Matilda.

But Tom was not there to talk fishing or hunting. He was there on the advice of his friends Ron and Matilda to seek a consultation on his wife, Beejay, who was newly diagnosed and just treated for malignant lymphoma. Hearing from Ron and Matilda of my lymphoma expertise, Tom wanted some help with a few questions.

There were enough questions and enough concerns that we were soon off in Tom's boat to see Beejay at their fish camp a few miles down the Niukluk. We arrived to a chorus of sled dogs and a waving Beejay, who greeted us in the friendly, somewhat shy, unaffected manner of the Inuit. Our conversation began easily among racks of drying salmon. I was invited in for a cozy cup of coffee with no need to remove my waders and boots. It was, after all, a fishing camp. We sat at her table and spoke of lymphoma with a basket of just-picked blueberries between us.

The camp was rustic, but it was not old-fashioned Inuit, with kayaks and sealskin clothing. It was twenty-first-century Inuit, with a generator, a chain saw, a computer, and a propane fridge. Beejay was just back from Anchorage, 600 miles away, after her second chemotherapy treatment. She was clearly tired but showing a lot of resolve and stoicism, also part of her Inuit heritage.

Her questions concerned the nature of her disease and the difficulty of her treatments. She understood her malignant lymphoma was a lethal threat. She knew of the necessity of chemotherapy. She wanted to know the cause of her disease. She asked if it would be passed on to her children. She wanted to know if the doctors in Anchorage at the Alaska Area Native Health Clinic were competent. She questioned whether she was getting the best and most effective treatment, or if she was being treated as an Inuit, as a second-class citizen. She puzzled over why she had to go to Anchorage for the next nine months since she was told after her last treatment that her scans were negative.

Lacking knowledge of the details, I gave her some hope, but I was not able to give her specific advice. I suggested that when I made it to Anchorage in four days, I would call her doctor, and then give her more specific advice. Hearing this and reading my uncertainty, Tom asked if I would like to speak to Beejay's doctor right then. Knowing we were 60 miles from Nome and 600 miles from Anchorage—in the middle of the Alaskan tundra without phone service—this seemed impossible. But Tom, the surprise techno geek, pulled out the latest and greatest satellite iridium phone. With this four-pound marvel hooked to twelve of Motorola's circulating satellites you could call anywhere on the planet any time. He used it to track his reindeer herd.

While I sat dumbfounded, Tom had me patched in and connected to Beejay's doctor in Anchorage. Then came an even bigger surprise. Amazingly, Dr. Dennis Beckworth was a first-class oncologist trained by us at the University of Arizona Cancer Center in Tucson. He had been one of the top trainees of our very own Dr. Miller. Just like that, it became old home week. With the speakerphone on Beejay's table, all the details, all the answers, came pouring out.

She had a diffuse large B-cell lymphoma. Her tumor biopsy had been studied on our Ventana instrument. The tumor was CD20-positive, and she was receiving the combination of chemotherapy (CHOP, a combination of four anti-cancer drugs) and anti-CD20-targeted therapy (Rituximab˙, the Roche/Genentech drug). And although now scan-negative, she was to receive six more courses of CHOP and Rituximab˙.

It became instantly clear that Beejay was receiving the best care on the planet. She had an outstanding oncologist who was giving her the latest miraculous anti-CD20-targeted therapy, a novel treatment based on the latest automation. Her prospect for cure was high. This was a harmonic convergence of the right information, the right doctor, and the right treatment. With a hearty thanks to Dr. Beckworth from all, we were back to chatting excitedly. Beejay's fear of substandard care vanished. She understood now that she was in good hands and was prepared to surrender to her care but for one doubt.

Why must she go to Anchorage for six more treatments if the tumor was gone? It was now August and that would mean going for a week every six weeks, much of it in the dead of winter and through the spring. Whereas the typical lower-forty-eight patient might get a babysitter and take a taxi to the nearby clinic, it was much more difficult for Beejay to chase the invisible. Imagine traveling 60 miles through a whiteout by snowmobile in the dead of winter at -60°F to the airport in Nome, then flying 600 miles to Anchorage for treatment. Getting there, getting treated, and getting back would be an arduous, risky, week-long process. Furthermore, Beejay—already weak—could not go alone; Tom needed to be her snowmobile driver and travel minder.

When they left the village, who would care for their children, their dogs, and their reindeer herd? That's right, their reindeer herd—which was a key component of their subsistence. Untended and unherded, the reindeer could be captured by wandering caribou herds. Undefended, they could be attacked by wolves. Then, how about in the spring? When they were gone, who would pick the fiddlehead ferns and gather the seagull eggs? Who would hunt the seal and render the seal oil? Without seal oil, how would the fiddleheads and the eggs be preserved for the next winter? The concerns went on and on. Who would cut the firewood? Who would mend the salmon nets? Who would maintain the snowmobile?

For Beejay, Tom, and their family, going to Anchorage another six to eight times was not just an inconvenience, it was a substantial threat to their subsistence. There were too many what-ifs to make chasing the invisible anything but a major burden and threat.

To overcome this major threat and to surrender to her demanding treatments at a great distance required a high degree of resolve and stoicism. This in turn required Tom and Beejay's total understanding of the nature of the beast, the need to sustain therapy to get the last cancer cell and overcome dormancy. Understanding all that, understanding the perils of winter travel, Beejay's final question was, "Why treat what is not there? If it's gone, why treat?"

My answer, as Dr. Miller had said before, was that to cure we must get the last malignant cell, including the one we couldn't see. To explain this to patients in Arizona, Dr. Miller had used the cockroach analogy, but in the cockroach-free tundra near the Arctic Circle, my analogy for Beejay was the mosquito. Beejay knew well the way of the Alaskan mosquito. She knew the swarms in the spring sprang from the dormant eggs surviving winter. She understood their dormancy, and so she came to see the wisdom in multiple rounds of therapy, however taxing to her and her family. She understood that to be cured she needed to chase the invisible, however great the cost. Our conversation came to a surprisingly reassuring conclusion. Now that Beejay fully understood the nature of the beast she was dealing with, she was all in and ready to surrender to her care.

She knew the way of the mosquito, the way of the bear, the way of the wolf. She knew how to keep them at bay. And now she knew the way of lymphoma and she knew how to escape its jaws. There was a new beast in her bestiary, but it was a beast understood and controllable. Her uncertainty over her doctor, of his diagnosis, and of her treatment, and of her need for action now behind her, she stood up, shook hands and said, "Thanks, I am good to go." So, a woman who had herded reindeer in the dead of winter in a gale at -60°F saw the task before her as surmountable.

Now for the musk-ox pot roast. It was two days later when Beejay and Tom brought to Ron and Matilda's fish camp the pot roast that Tom had shot and Beejay had prepared, along with Yukon potatoes from her garden, and a blueberry pie made from the basket of blueberries on her table. We all sat down to a great feast worthy of Julia Child and James Beard. Besides the sumptuousness of the roast and the delicacy of the pie, the real pleasure was the revelry. It was not only the pleasure of the bounty of the tundra, but the good cheer and the genuine enjoyment of the moment. Joy in the moment. The talk was not of lymphoma or therapy, but of the silver run, the huckleberry harvest, the stalking of the musk ox, the hunting of moose, and the herding of reindeer.

No physician ever received a finer reward for a house call than that day with a musk-ox pot roast, a blueberry pie, and revelry. Twelve years later, and for the twenty-third time, I waylaid myself on the Niukluk and visited Beejay and Tom at their fish camp. Beejay and I would again pose for our annual you-must-be-cured photo after a cup of coffee, and we spoke of the way of the salmon, the way of the wolf, and the way of the mosquito.

And so it is with the best medicine that normalcy intervenes, revelry returns, and subsistence, in all its Alaskan abundance and resolve, goes on unconstrained by a passing beast.

Energized by the excitement of the practice of medicine, Mom and I returned to stories of the business. It was then painful to recollect that, although my team had a fabulous transformative product, what we didn't have was a market. That, we had to make from scratch.

10.

Selling the Future

INVENTORS INVARIABLY BELIEVE WHEN THEIR creation is built, the job is done. The hard part is over. All that is left is to sell what is an obviously great product. "Build it and they will come," is their belief. As it turns out, that belief is false. The self-assured, high-minded inventor does not understand that much remains to be done. The inventors, for all their brilliance, have created something valuable—a product—but what they have not created is a market. Just because you have a light bulb doesn't mean you have an illuminated city. Just because you have a product to sell doesn't mean you have a customer to buy it. Why would a customer buy a product never seen, to produce results never seen, at prices never seen? It's new. It's expensive. It's risky.

Inventors don't know what they don't know. But they soon learn that making a market will involve just as much creativity and human effort as the original invention. It will require new forms of intelligence: social intelligence, cultural intelligence, knowledge of marketing methods, something called salesmanship, and something called tech support.

It turns out that making a market involves creative selling and a total commitment to customer support. You have to find 'em, convince 'em, sell 'em, support 'em, and finally love 'em to death. Good luck doing that with a PhD scientist or engineer. So we began the next phase by hiring new talent in marketing, sales, and tech support. And this phase was to prove every bit as arduous and demanding of creativity as the inventive phase.

The first step for our new marketing and sales team was to call attention to our product at national pathology and lab medicine meetings. With the offering of a free box lunch, potential customers, including pathologists and technicians, were lured into a large conference room to see our newborn, to marvel at the sleek ready-to-use automated instrument.

Our sales manager gave a twenty-minute demonstration using a few barcoded slides. It was a bit like one of Julia Child's cooking shows on PBS. There was a lot of chatter, a bit of prep (e.g. placing the barcode on a slide), a flourish with the slide popped in the oven, blinking lights on the control panel, and then a tray of previously cooked slides was brought to a multi-headed microscope for all to see the baked goodies. On the wall, there were a couple of big signs that read, *Seeing is believing; You push the button, we do the rest.* And, *Send your tech home early.*

It was interactive, it was lively, it was a free lunch. Standing in the corner, I thought how easy selling could be, but I was soon brought back to earth. When the fun was over, we stood by the door, hearing the participants.

"Wow, impressive. But for that kind of money I could hire two more techs."

"My tech already does a great job. I'll hire another and save money to boot."

"Why pay a vendor for saltwater solutions that we already make for nothing? I don't need another vendor in my life."

"So what about that prepackaged DAB carcinogen? My tech doesn't mind the glove-and-gown routine."

"We send all our tough cases out to the university. I don't feel comfortable taking on a whole new way of thinking. This involves a lot of new lingo, words like immunohistochemistry. None of which we had in med school."

"There is no billing code for IHC. Why would I spend money to lose money?"

"Why would I want to buy an instrument for which I have no budget to produce a test for which there is no compensation?"

"If I buy this contraption, I will have new maintenance and repair costs. My tech doesn't require maintenance and repair."

"Okay, I get the tractor benefit—I just worry about the gas. Once we're hooked, they can jack up the prices and take us to the cleaners."

And so we were to learn from our customers. We learned they were inclined to a free lunch; they were inclined to be entertained but disinclined to buy. They had too much uncertainty, imagined too many problems. This was our clearly expressed voice of the customer (VOC). The VOC was the marketeer's voice of reality. The VOC was the unmistakable voice of the market, and our VOC was unequivocal—you have a technology searching for a market; you are ahead of your time. This might fly at the university but not at the community lab, said the community MDs. And the university academics said, "We are happy as the regional masters of IHC. We are happy to be the exalted consultant."

The VOC was saying, "No." So should we pack it up and go home? After all, the customers are always right, aren't they?

Thinking back to Henry Ford and Steve Jobs, the answer was no. Sometimes the VOC is right, and sometimes it's wrong. When Henry Ford offered a horseman a car, he said he preferred a faster horse, and when Steve Jobs first offered a smartphone, the users—already owning most of the components separately—dismissed it as an unwanted confection. What Ford, Jobs, and eventually we learned from subsequent success was that the early VOC is imperfect, requiring careful qualification. When the VOC speaks to product refinement, it is valuable, but when it comes to transformative products, it is not.

In retrospect, our early VOC experience needed to be qualified. We would now say that was the voice of the later adopters. Fortunately, the voice we came to hear and depend on was more imaginative, and future-seeing. This was also a VOC, but what we came to call the *voice of the cognoscenti.* Out of the more than two hundred VOCs we heard at the demos, there were just a few—four to five—who got it. They saw not just the future, but the immediacy of the future. They were the rare, hard-to-find, natural early adopters, the first in the neighborhood to buy a car or a smartphone. In this category of the early-adopter cognoscenti were three who were to become our first customers, and on whom we were to bet the whole enterprise.

They were Dr. Gist Farr (remember him from Letterman?), now at the Ochsner Clinic (the first in), and then Dr. Ray Tubbs at the Cleveland Clinic, then Dr. Pat Roche at the Mayo Clinic. They each ran labs at large, famous private clinics. They had national and international reputations, serving as referral centers, practicing medicine at the highest levels, often taking on the toughest medical patients, as I was doing in Arizona. They had large practices involving thousands of patients, and they were most in need of automation to assist. They needed to tackle scale.

We fit their need to serve many and to serve better. We fit their need for large scale. But they ultimately gave us more than just the cash for instruments. They were to give us our marketing narrative. From them, we came to understand we were not just selling instruments and tests; we were selling the practice of medicine. We were selling the ability to improve diagnostic accuracy and patient care. The value lay in the pathologist achieving greater diagnostic accuracy, and the lab tech delivering timelier and more reliable results without physical exhaustion. The value lay in the productivity of the techs, and their becoming the masters of an automated delivery system rather than handmaidens to the bucket brigade. The value also lay in eliminating the carcinogenic threat and the glove-and-gown experience.

These were all values our sales force could believe in, demonstrate, and sell to. The cognoscenti had given us our selling path. From then on, we were not just selling the car. We were selling the driving experience.

Besides better medicine, the cognoscenti took us to school on another key element of making a market—service and support. Once a clinic or a hospital began running on our device, we quickly learned reliability was the top priority. A hospital runs 24/7, and any downtime is a catastrophe. For them, the immediacy and certainty of technical support was critical. We used to say, "If the customer sneezes, we get pneumonia."

The glory of innovation and the thrill of selling vanish in the shadow of downtime. Owning this problem was essential and exhausting. In fact, it was a good thing we only sold six instruments in 1991; if we had sold sixty, we would have gone bankrupt given the enormous cost of customer support. In particular their needs were educational as all the instrument-rendered results were new to medicine and not yet taught in medical schools. In the end, our total commitment to support, our zeal in owning all the problems, is what established our reputation and our market.

We survived that first critical year because we were obsessed with staying close to the customer. It was management by proximity. It was a combination of service visits and frequent phone calls. It was listening and acting with urgency. Each member of the leadership team was assigned one of the first six. I was assigned Dr. Ray Tubbs at the Cleveland Clinic. I had my hands full with Ray. He was out to transform the Cleveland Clinic lab, and the medical practice, and he was obsessed with new diagnostic tests and new refinements. He was also obsessed with total reliability and the need to adjust. He was quick to call me anytime, anywhere, including at home. There were many calls for assistance. I recall one particular exchange.

My home phone was ringing off the hook. It was Ray, and he was in a rage. With hardly a hello, he launched into a blistering tirade. Rising from bed, blearily, I focused on the clock. It was 4:30 a.m. Ray was never time constrained, and besides, it was 6:30 a.m. in Cleveland. Despite the time, I knew this must be important and must be dealt with. I interrupted, "Ray, this sounds serious. Let's get to the bottom of it. But if you don't mind, let me hang up and call you right back."

Ray paused. "Sorry, are you alright?"

"Yeah," I said. "It's just that I can't do this standing buck naked."

Two minutes later we were reconnected. "Okay, Ray, I'm ready for action."

"First," Ray said, "I have a question. What's the difference between naked and buck naked?"

"Don't you know?" I responded. "It's a pair of socks. I hate sleeping with cold feet." We had a good laugh, and then dove into our problem.

When I look back, making a market meant much more than selling. It meant attention to service and support, and sometimes it meant getting up early and standing buck naked to face your challenges.

Gist Farr, Ray Tubbs, and Pat Roche were to become much more than customers; they were to become scientific advisers to Ventana for the next twenty years. Pat was to be even more integral, as he became a key Ventana senior scientist, directing our antibody effort and our link to pharma. While Ray didn't become an employee, he was to go on informing our future.

Ray's effort to bring DNA and RNA tests known as in-situ hybridization (ISH) assays to the standard hospital microscope for everyone to see produced a major creative breakthrough with major consequences for patients and for our business. He combined efforts with Nanoprobes Inc. to create an automated single-gene test for the HER2 gene based on silver-particle nanotechnology. He employed a process akin to silver-grain black-and-white photography. By this means, in a process we were to call silver in-situ hybridization (SISH), he was able to detect and light up the two HER2 genes, one from the mom and one from the dad, in every cell in a tissue biopsy. He could easily see those two genes out of a denominator of 60,000 genes, 30,000 from the mom and 30,000 from the dad. Ray picking out these two genes was the equivalent of Perceval Lowell picking out Pluto in the night sky. For both, the key was a new tool: fine-grain silver photography.

On the heels of this remarkable feat, I got another unscheduled, excited phone call from Ray. He was over-the-moon excited; it was as if he were Lowell himself and had just discovered Pluto. He asked me to get to Cleveland as soon as possible.

A few days on, I sat across from him at his microscope. He explained that he had added another wrinkle to enhance his creation. He followed his SISH HER2 gene assay with a protein HER2 assay by IHC, so both the gene and the protein could be seen at once. You could see both the pathologic gene amplification and the consequent increase in protein. As he said, we could now see cause and effect.

In that moment, on that crisp, cold December morning in Cleveland in 2001, knee-to-knee with Ray at the microscope, I was to see what had never been seen before in a standard light microscope. I saw a tissue biopsy of invasive breast carcinoma showing an amplification of more than twenty HER2 genes per cancer cell and a massive increase in HER2 protein in the same cancer cells. These cancer cells had ten times the growth impetus of normal cells. No wonder they had the capacity to kill the patient. Looking with Ray, I too saw cause and effect. I too saw the mechanism of disease and the target for anti-HER2 therapy. And we both realized the implication that—thanks to automation—this could be done anywhere on the planet. As it turned out, this was to be one reason the Swiss, with their miracle anti-HER2 drug, Herceptin*, were to come calling on Ventana in 2007. Ray was, by that measure, living in the future by creating it.

What we saw on that day in Cleveland was precisely what Gaddafi saw eight years later in 2009 when he sat down knee-to-knee with our Libyan MD (see Fig. 1). Thanks to Roche, the Swiss pharmaceutical company with a major diagnostics unit, Ray's mission of globalization was to be fully realized.

We learned a lot from those first three customers. We learned of the demand and requirements to grow the practice of medicine at the top medical clinics. We learned what it took to supply and support. We learned our narrative from the three, but one swallow does not a spring make, and three customers do not a business make.

It was time to go beyond the voice of the cognoscenti to tackle the painful voice of the customer we heard earlier. It was time to find and persuade the late adopters to join the future. It was time to confront their problems, including the lack of a capital budget, a lack of test compensation, and a lack of comfort with the new science of immunohistochemistry, in-situ hybridization, and automation. It was time to sell tractors to horse farmers who just wanted a faster horse. It was time to solve Henry Ford's problem.

The architect of this next major effort to reach every farmer and universalize sales was our CEO, Chris Gleeson. Chris was a world-class salesman who was hired to bring us to commercial success. His task was to articulate our sales strategy, create our commercial blueprint, and help us achieve widespread adoption.

Chris launched his plan with two dramatic gestures. First, he brought on a team of world-class sales team leaders, including Hany Massarany, Jim LaFrance, Jack Phillips, Steve Hagen and Pete Bantock.

Second, they created a new sales paradigm. At the plant in Tucson, they built a gleaming new lab of the future. It was fully outfitted with our latest automated instruments and stocked with all of our latest chemistries, including more than a hundred IHC protein assays and in-situ hybridization tests (ISH) for DNA and RNA. It also had a bank of clinical cases demonstrating the latest diagnosis-changing cases.

Gleeson and team then brought the skeptical, late adopters to Tucson to spend several days in our lab of the future. They brought along some of their own tissue blocks, so they could generate their own results on the spot. The Ventana team ushered them into the future. They gave them a day in a diagnostic Disneyland. They let them touch and feel the future and made them want to bring it home with them.

They did what Thomas Edison did in 1880. A hundred years before Chris, Edison had the same problem. He had a product, the incandescent light bulb. He even had his own power-plant electricity generator and his own grid. But what he did not have was a way to get every town in America to buy the system. It was too expensive, too complicated, and too unfamiliar. Small-town America had no budget for building a power plant. It had no budget to build a distribution system, and besides, it already had illumination by kerosene, candle, and gaslight.

To solve his adoption problem, Edison used his Wall Street capital to create a demonstration project in Menlo Park, New Jersey. He opened for public view his own two-city-block electrified laboratory and the adjacent houses and streets (Stross). This gave physical form to the new incandescent utopia. It demonstrated a brighter, safer, literally enlightened future. It showed Everytown, USA, as brighter, safer, cleaner, and available for the asking, or more specifically, for the buying. The commercialization was then driven by bringing town officials and politicians by rail to Menlo Park to create the enthusiasm. As it turned out, their seeing was indeed believing, and so a small, lighted village ushered in the electrification of a nation and a planet.

Chris's "lab of the future" in Tucson was the equivalent of Edison's electrified village in New Jersey. They both enabled prospective customers to make physical contact with the transformative product. It gave them physical proximity. Chris and team let the horse farmer not only see the tractor, but also drive it. And as we added the element of real-time medical cases, they could see they would be improving their practices back home. As with Edison, the idea was for the potential customer to experience the transformative power and to make them understand if they brought this to their hospital, they would be the pioneers. After that, all Chris and team had to do was throw in a few after-hours margaritas, maybe a round of golf, and a stuffed poblano pepper or two, and their success rate exceeded 90 percent. The rest was just finding money and working budgets.

Subsequently, seeking to move more potential customers into the future, Chris and team developed another powerful method. This was a go-to-the-customer outreach approach whereby a salesperson would drop off an instrument on loan to play with for thirty days. After a fifteen-minute setup and training, the users were usually addicted within hours. Again, about 90 percent of the time, the box stayed put. In some cases, thirty days turned into thirty years. And thirty years on, these were the methods that led us down the path to selling more than twelve thousand instruments and running tests for twenty million patients per annum.

From my frequent interactions with them, Mom came to know Gist, Ray, Pat and Chris well. As we recollected their many contributions, she included them in her pantheon of like souls. As she remarked to me, "They not only lived in the future; they created it."

11.

Seabiscuit and Barking Seals

IN 1996, WE HAD An invention transformed into a product of proven utility, but what we didn't have was a market. We did not have a national supply and support system equivalent to Edison's power grid. We proved we could sell to individuals, but to make it to every hospital, in every city in the country, we needed something else we didn't have—Wall Street capital.

To go everywhere, to change the practice of medicine, to universalize the change would require going beyond the tens of millions of dollars already invested to hundreds of millions. It meant going from the private control in our hands to the demands and uncertainties of public control. However, for a small startup tech company like us, situated off the tech map at the edge of the known universe, to go public with an initial public offering (IPO) on Wall Street was a near impossibility.

For one thing, our company was one of the first in Tucson to successfully attempt it. The Arizona economy was known for its five Cs: copper, cotton, citrus, cattle, and climate. There was no substantive biotech industry. What Arizona did have was a Science I university, the University of Arizona, with an abundance of science and engineering talent and a top-shelf medical school. The state had the potential for a sixth *C*, the cerebral cortex, which drives knowledge-based industry, but nothing had garnered Wall Street's attention before.

To invest hard-earned, retirement-needed cash in an unknown startup, with an unknown invention, of unknown economic consequence, in a far-off unknown place the public needed reassurances, which came from analysts at Wall Street investment firms. The analysts were professional bookies who knew the racetrack and knew the horses. In the risky business of betting on the unknown, they calculated the odds. They knew horseflesh, and they knew a winner when they saw one. By that calculus, the medical device–knowledgeable bookies could see the promise, but for them to back us would be like choosing to invest in an undersized, runty, unpredictable horse known as Seabiscuit, when everyone else could see that Man o' War was a physically superior horse and a sure bet. But as every professional bookie knows, more money is made on the risky bets than sure things. Provided, of course, the runt comes through.

Besides the many unknown risks we presented, there were known risks adding to the unlikeliness of our success. First was the enormous effort required to make it into the practice of medicine with a new device. To change medicine, which by nature is highly conservative, would require elaborate proof of safety and efficacy and the imprimatur of the FDA to assure the change was appropriate. The costs of the requisite medical clinical studies necessary to please medical and regulatory skeptics would be predictably enormous. Second, even if we achieved medical proof of safety and efficacy as required by the FDA and practitioners, there was yet another formidable constraint—the economics of diagnostics, which were well known to have a problem with undervaluation. It was said diagnostics were pennies on the pharma dollar. Because of these factors it was rational to conclude our venture would cost a fortune and never achieve economic success.

Given this level of skepticism, how were these dismissive analysts to be won over? What would convince them that dumping capital into a traditionally undervalued field with historic low economic gain would pay off? We had to wonder not just what but also who would convince them to take the risk.

Enter Jack Schuler, the critical *who*. He was to become our chief persuader to Wall Street and to other major institutional investors. He was not the only factor, but he was a major contributor in convincing the analysts ours was a horse that would win, and that the race would be thrilling and profitable.

Jack became the de-risker in chief in the eyes of the analysts and investment bankers. Why such influence? Because Jack, as the former CEO and president of Abbott Labs, had twenty-five years of experience in the medical device industry. He was a driving force in making Abbott the premier American diagnostic company in laboratory medicine. Wall Street held him in high regard for his many accomplishments. Starting on the R & D side of medical devices, he had successfully gone from invention, to product, to FDA approval, to making a market with numerous well-known diagnostics. He had done this not only in the US market but also globally. In his previous position at Texas Instruments, he famously—with great energy and intelligence—opened the Japanese market to US instruments by invoking US congressional passions and assistance.

Much later, on the heels of his Abbott fame, Jack left for greener pastures, joining John Patience (JP) in co-founding Crabtree Ventures, a medical venture-capital company out of Chicago. Soon thereafter, Jack became board chairman of Ventana and JP the vice chair. At that point, every bookie on the street knew this Seabiscuit was a horse worth betting on. They may not have been completely sure of the horse or the pasture it was in, but they sure knew the jockey. Bring on the race.

Having won over the Wall Street investors, the IPO was set up for six weeks hence with one critical step in between—the roadshow. The roadshow entails traveling city to city to pre-sell the IPO. It is the opportunity for institutional investors like retirement funds to get in early and, in doing so, to ensure an early IPO success. Jack was also instrumental in that process, explaining how automation would re-valuate the pathology lab and how the business would be profitable. As he appeared before the likes of the Wisconsin teachers' retirement fund, he explained our business model as the "razor-razorblade" approach, with the automated instrument as the razor and the antibody tests as the blades. We sold the razor cheap and the razor blades at great margins. He explained easily how our chemistry was microscope-readable, how we were able to make the otherwise invisible cells visible through attached dyes and, as a result, raise the bar on accurate diagnosis.

He explained how our device could go anywhere in the world; all that was needed was an electrical outlet and a standard microscope. These simple requirements meant our market was huge. As the ever-charismatic persuader in chief, Jack was the sharp cutting edge to our razor-razorblade business model. And as the driving force on our board, Jack always had his foot on the accelerator, leaving the rest of us to pump the brakes.

Having won over the institutional investors, the IPO went through on July 3, 1996, selling three million shares at $10 a share. With the added tens of millions, we had the means to go beyond the university lab to the community lab, and to go beyond the local to the national. We now had the means to universalize. In a manner Adam Smith would find familiar and admirable in his equation of the benefit of capitalism, we had turned an invention into a useful product that benefited patients and drew on public funds, which also benefited investors like the Wisconsin teachers' retirement fund. Tom Edison would also find familiar the equation from invention to product to universal utility through Wall Street alliance.

Smith and Edison would agree a new enterprise is risky business, but risk is where improvement and gain lie, so bring it on.

Imagine taking a final exam in a tough subject like algebra or geometry every three months for twelve years. It might turn you into an English major.

As tough as it was, we took those exams, known as shareholder conference calls, forty-eight times over twelve years on NASDAQ from 1996 to 2008. That was forty-eight quarterly reports filed and addressed on telephone conference calls with analysts and shareholders, both institutional and individual. The calls, our oral exams, were meant to answer a key question. Did we meet expectations? Expectations were based on results the analysts had forecast months before, laying out their calculations for growth of the business and for quarterly revenue.

Our quarterly grade was not the usual grade school A, B, C, D, or F. Rather it was pass/fail. *A* if we met expectations and *F* if we didn't. As it turned out, we met expectations forty-eight times in a row, sometimes by the skin of our teeth, and sometimes resoundingly. As rosy as that sounds, excellence was, as any A student will attest, demanding and difficult to sustain. We worked hard on constant contact with the analysts to keep expectations realistic. We were careful to under-promise and over-deliver.

Much has been criticized about the short-term quarterly mentality, but it set our pace. It became a part of our routine. It brought us discipline and the rigors of financial analysis. Yet forty-eight times also instilled a mindset that we were running a marathon, not a sprint, and persistence was our mantra.

It is said that the stock market is driven by greed and fear. It is, above all else, the land of acquisitiveness and avarice, as our later experience with investment bankers taught us. That pejorative comes from the periodic excess of the Street, like the tech-bubble burst of 2000 or the great collapse in 2008 following the systemic failure of securitized high-risk mortgages. Those failures are the consequence of hype and exaggerated claims used to drive up share value and realize unfounded gain. In 2000, it was overvaluing the promise of tech companies before they even had products or viable businesses. In 2008, it was the Street falsely legitimizing illegitimate mortgages. It was reveling in the rise and ignoring the risk. It was insider trading and frontend skimming. Worst of all, it was hiding the truth.

We took the opposite approach. It was not exaggerated claims, but evidence based. It was instruments sold, revenue earned, customers pleased. It was observable and measurable. The customer experience could be observed firsthand. It was evidence gained by proximity to the customer and transparency of the user experience. It was about producing value for the customer and thereby value to the investors. Greed was out of the picture. It was old-fashioned long-term capital gain based on value creation—not hype.

As for the latter part of the greed-and-fear equation, we did experience periodic fear of failure on the part of the analysts and institutions. Our constant dialogue with them tempered the tendency toward an "irrational exuberance" described by Federal Reserve Chairman Alan Greenspan, and this generally brought about realistic expectations. But sometimes that same proximity and transparency invoked skepticism. Even though our revenue and growth goals were met quarterly, the analysts were always in fear of future failure. For example, an analyst hearing an FDA approval was delayed, or about out-of-box failure of instruments, or about customer backorders, could become alarmed if not assured a solution was forthcoming. Consequently, the now-skeptical analyst could downgrade future expectations. Even one cautionary downgrade by just one analyst could produce a chain reaction in what we called the "barking-seal effect." One seal in a colony of hundreds on a beach might see a shark fin in the distant sea. The one begins barking and soon the entire colony is a-bark—not because they too see a fin, but because the other seals are barking.

And so it was, once even one analyst barked, the others would soon panic and join the chorus. It quickly turned into what Greenspan might call "exaggerated skepticism." This is especially common over the prospects of small startup companies, since nine out of ten fail eventually. Out of that knowledge, even a rumor of difficulty can lead to the selling of shares, and then selling begets selling.

Adding to the commotion, there were often individuals selling short. That is, betting the share price would dip and selling shares they didn't own with the expectation they could buy them cheaper before the transaction closed. As periodically happened to us, these individuals, known as shorts, sometimes ballooned in number. The shorts would go into a frenzy of short betting when they perceived difficulty in the future of the company or the marketplace. Imagine in horse racing if there was the ability to bet on which horse was certain to lose. If so, and you saw a horse with a limp, you would have a sure bet to win on a loss. Similarly, the shorts can see a limp in a company and have a sure bet on a downturn, as happened in 2008 when billions were won shorting companies that were heavily into securitized high-risk mortgages like Lehman Brothers. Some saw the limp and won on the ultimate predictable failure of these companies.

This state of exaggerated skepticism and short selling can lead to a vicious downward cycle. In our case, this powerful tide was stemmed when John Patience, and Jack Schuler bought a significant number of shares, restoring confidence in the enterprise. After all, if the lead investors are buying, there may be an opportunity, following an old Wall Street adage, "Buy good companies on bad news."

And so, in the midst of this rising clamor, this din of barking seals, Patience and Schuler exercised their decisive action. By buying aggressively, they demonstrated their personal confidence in the enterprise. By doing so, the two, as highly regarded seals, quieted the colony. Perhaps it wasn't a shark after all; perhaps it was just a dolphin. Ho-hum.

The personal commitment and daring of Patience and Schuler helped all recalculate the risk-to-gain ratio, and the barking colony settled into a quiet night's sleep ashore. And so it was by keeping our attention on the development and refinement of our instruments, and by supporting our customers, that we came to be a reliable, rising star on NASDAQ. We focused on adding value to our customers, and in time we were able to pass that value on to our stalwart investors. This old-fashioned system of long-term capitalism was to benefit many, and greed and fear had nothing to do with it.

Our plan was not a three-year effort with a three-to-five-times return on investment (ROI). Our plan was to keep inventing and building until we changed the practice of medicine, period. Money was not our end point; it was our enabler.

Thanks to the impact of our new capital, we steadily grew our market and pleased Wall Street by increasing our sales by double digits.

As pleased as the Street was, there were underlying difficulties. Namely, creating the national sales and support teams, growing R & D, and building out manufacturing with a new physical plant was costing us an alarming amount.

Our operational costs were eating us alive to the tune of $2 million a quarter. Adding up the then eight years of operational costs, we were down $48 million, with capital spent.

JP and I were in the hallway about to enter the boardroom to report another operational cost of $4 million. But before we stepped into the room, JP stopped.

"Are you all right?" JP was looking hard at me.

"No," I replied.

"What's wrong?"

"I think I may be sick."

"Is it a virus?'

"No, I'm having an anxiety attack. I can't take it anymore. I can't take more capital expenses and debt. I can't take that we have spent so much. I can't face the directors. I can't face the shareholders. I keep thinking of shareholders like the retired schoolteacher in Wisconsin whose retirement fund is invested in us. We cannot continue to take her money, their money, and turn it into losses."

"Take it easy," JP said. "Get a grip. The way we're spending money, we're going to make a *lot* of money." He placed a reassuring hand on my shoulder.

"That is a ridiculous, absurd, delusional statement! You can't win by losing," I said. "Now I'm even more upset."

"Why is that?" JP pressed.

"Because you're supposed to be the strictly objective, totally analytical, linear-thinking financial analyst. I am the pie-in-the-sky, blue-sky, non-linear medical guy. You are scaring the hell out of me. How could we possibly make money given the hole we're in?"

"All right," JP said. "Let me explain how this capitalism thing works. It is true we are down forty-eight million, but that is not money lost, that's money invested. That's not debt. It's equity, not cash burned. That is capital invested to create value. It's long-term capital devoted to solving problems and making progress. That teacher in Wisconsin has not lost her money. She has invested in creating new value so her pension will grow, not shrink. That teacher's retirement fund has equity. That teacher owns the upside as we grow and realize profits to be shared as dividends and increased share value. That teacher understands you have to spend money to make money. She is going to ride the economic gain from here."

"Thanks for the Adam Smith sermon, but we are still forty-eight million in the hole," I insisted. "And your statement that the way we're losing money means we're going to make money remains delusional."

"It's not delusional, and here's why. My prediction is based on fact, not fallacy."

"Really, what are you smoking?"

"True, we are down forty-eight million, but look at what we have created, how our automation and chemistry are transforming medicine. You need to understand the medical device business. It's a cycle. First you invest, then you build, then you sell, then you support, then you transform, and then—lastly—you profit. It's a six-step process and we are just now moving through step five. Predictably, stage six will follow."

"Honest to God, are you dreaming this up?"

"No." JP stuck to his guns. "Just look at the Cleveland Clinic. We have completely transformed their practice. We have made it to step five with them. All of their reports include our chemistry now. Their oncologists have timely results on every patient. They are running on our instruments every day. They have moved completely from the horse to the tractor, and we supply the tractor."

"Okay, I hear you, but honestly every month we get calls about their reliability problems."

"Right. They've given up the horse and they want to run the tractor 24/7. Great. Perfect. Now we invest in reliability and keep them running at all costs."

"Oh great," I retorted. "More losses."

"No. Greater reliability, greater impact, greater return on investment. Here's the way I see it: when they commit to drive our tractor, we commit to zero downtime. We should take the view that when they sneeze, we get pneumonia. We invest all we have now in support. Then we sell the total solution."

"Good. Spending more money." I was still not convinced. "How much cash does the Wisconsin teachers' retirement fund have on hand?"

"Stop. Here is the part you must get. We have transformed the Cleveland Clinic. Our proof case is established. Our model is set.

Now we just turn every lab, in every hospital, in every city, in every country into the Cleveland Clinic. And then, bingo, our investment comes back as profit, and that is how capitalism works. We just reassure the teacher in Wisconsin her economic gain merely awaits our fulfilling the plan. So buck up; don't throw up. Be confident and remember, the way we're losing, we're sure to win. That's not being Pollyanna; that's being rational and factual."

Fast-forward to the board meeting. I lightened the talk of heavy costs with an account of our scientific and medical progress, including a testimonial from the Cleveland Clinic about how we were improving their practice and benefiting individual patients. Presentation made, confidence regained, board resolved to keep on. Funny how a veneer of confidence can cover a sea of uncertainty. Funny how a true friend and colleague can supply the veneer just in time and save the day.

Mom, who had taught us to see and take on danger and to not be consumed by fright, liked this story. She liked JP's resolve and confidence. She liked that JP and I were succeeding by alliance.

12.

All In

WITH TIME, BUSINESS GREW AS our customers looked to us to fulfill their ever-increasing tissue diagnostic needs. The burgeoning field of targeted, personalized cancer therapy was calling for more and more companion-diagnostic tools to determine which therapies would be most effective for individual patients, and our customers' lab volumes grew accordingly.

In the process, we soon learned it was not enough to invent it, to make it, to sell it, and to support it. You had to go back and refine and improve. You had to make the instrument easier to use and more reliable. To that end, we adopted the mantra, "Never stop refining; never stop inventing." To realize this aspiration, we devoted ourselves to building a culture of innovation, refinement and strict accountability. And this applied to all employees of every rank and file. They had battled with us and would celebrate our collective victory.

It was the silent tears streaming down the cheeks of one of our employees, Norma Maughan (née Aguilar) at 9 a.m. on July 12, 2003, that came to personify the strong inclusive culture we had built. On that day, we were in New York City to ring the opening bell at the NASDAQ to call attention to our rising-star status on the Wall Street exchange.

As we stood on the platform for the ceremony, there was great excitement among the thirty Ventana employees present. This was the moment that affirmed our success as an enterprise. This was the culmination of over a decade of hard work. This was recognition of the importance of our products and our business methods. This was the stamp of approval from the Wall Street analysts, the institutional investors, and the US Securities and Exchange Commission (SEC). We were in high capitalistic clover.

After the ringing of the bell, there was an eruption of clapping, hand shaking and hugging. As I turned to Norma, her cheeks were damp. Concerned, I asked if she was all right.

"Oh yes, yes," she said. "I am over the moon. I am living the American Dream!" As it turned out, these were tears of joy.

On that unforgettable day, Norma was there on the platform not as a senior VP or project manager of Ventana. She was not from the top brass. She was there because she was an outstanding employee and a recognized cultural hero.

Norma was the dedicated, driven employee who was every employer's dream. She had come from Guadalajara, Mexico, to Tucson as the first of her family to attend college. She had come to Ventana taking a lower-level starting job in reagent packaging and shipping.

But Norma, as a force of nature like so many diligent and determined immigrants in the US, a country of immigrants, was out to prove herself through hard work. Norma strongly identified with the company's mission and totally devoted herself to that purpose. She took the view that delivering the product was just as important as inventing the product. Within three years, she became a team leader in test-kit packaging. She valued her work as vital, and she assumed complete, personal ownership of every detail and difficulty in that function. It was her commitment and work ethic that earned Norma a place on the platform.

Later that day, when I asked Norma about the American Dream, she said, "I came from a very poor family in rural Mexico. As one of ten children, I had to walk an hour and a half to school through the cornfields. We were so poor that sometimes there was not enough food, and the older children skipped meals so the younger ones could eat. But I have found happiness in America. I have fully developed my capabilities, and I am here in New York City at NASDAQ in front of the camera being recognized for my work. This for me is a dream come true!"

Not then, because we were all having too much fun, but sometime later I reflected on Norma's version of the American Dream. I was struck by how she defined her dream as attaining fulfillment by developing her capabilities, applying them to a higher purpose, and being recognized and rewarded.

Years later, when I came again to reflect on Norma's version of the American Dream, I became curious if there was a more formal definition. To my surprise, I found the phrase was coined in 1931 by James Truslow Adams in his book, *The Epic of America*, written amid the Great Depression. As he defined it, the American Dream was not about becoming rich and famous; it was about the opportunity to live your life to its fullest potential and being appreciated for who you are as an individual, not because of your type or rank or circumstances of birth.

It sounded a lot like Thomas Jefferson writing the Declaration of Independence and declaring a right for all to life, liberty and *the pursuit of happiness.*

Jefferson didn't mention rich and famous, nor did Norma on that fateful day. Norma's dream was not first of riches and fame but of personal fulfillment and individual growth and recognition. She welled up that day over hard-earned recognition of her talents and effort. As she saw it, the company brought her to New York City for the whole world to see.

Norma's fulfillment came from being given a job with a purpose, a chance to enhance her talents, and an opportunity to demonstrate her value and achieve recognition. By these measures, Norma was not just living the American Dream—she *was* the American Dream. Norma was not just a product of the culture. She was the culture.

And so, as we grew over the years, we were to find and nurture the Norma equivalents in every department and every function. As it turns out, a company with a thousand Normas is a remarkable, productive, fulfilled company, and riches and fame are the lesser rewards. When dreaming is connected to doing, your products are not only imagined, but delivered.

At this writing, twenty years later, Norma is the senior manager of instrument assembly with forty employees in her charge. Norma reminds us all of the virtue underlying the American Dream.

Besides Norma, there were many more like-minded immigrants, altogether one hundred and fifty from thirty countries who enhanced our culture.

There was Junshan Hao from China, Lidija Pestic-Dragovich from Serbia, Hiro Nitta from Japan, and Noemi Sebastiao from Canada. They each came from disadvantage. Each of them came to the US seeking a better life, and all of them dealt with their disadvantages by acquiring new skills and working tirelessly to succeed. They responded to disadvantage and discomfort by taking action.

Over time, through persistence and merit, they each succeeded. Junshan as a key chemist in our operations group, solving a myriad of technical problems; Lidija as a top scientist heading our pharma-connected companion-diagnostics scientific group; and Hiro as the lead scientist in my own Ventana lab for more than twenty years. It was Hiro who developed the dual-labeled HER2 test later seen by Gaddafi. It was his effort and that test that received FDA approval and drew Roche's attention, resulting in the Swiss acquisition.

Noemi, of Portuguese descent, who was trained as a medical technologist, became the head of our technical support group after she was named on one of the most important patents in our history. She was called out by name as an inventor, along with Kimberly Christiansen, a mechanical engineer, and Ethel McCrae, a technologist of Native American descent. Their invention became the foundation for our second- and third-generation instruments. Noemi traveled the world in technical support and is distinguished by having delivered and installed one of our farthest-flung instruments, in Umtata, South Africa, near Nelson Mandela's native village.

Along with Norma, these individuals and many others like them gave us a culture rich in diverse immigrant backgrounds steeped in self-discipline, determination, and a drive for success. As they each became American citizens, they were to live the American Dream. Junshan, for example, proudly has a son who became a neurosurgeon.

When I look back, the culture was not just me; it was a phalanx of like-minded, self-made individuals. Our culture, as they defined it, was driven by a strong desire to overcome disadvantage by acquiring new skills. My part was to unify the effort by giving them a common purpose.

From the perspective of modern-day immigration policy, it is important to recognize these five came here before they achieved advanced degrees, but they contributed mightily because they arrived loaded with the most important attribute of all—motivation.

When I reflect on where that vibrant culture personified by Norma came from, several factors stand out as the building blocks of our corporate culture.

First, as the founder, as the original salesman and persuader, I understood from the beginning that we needed to firmly establish the company's belief system. I needed for everyone involved to understand the *why*. I needed for all of them, like Catherine and Dr. Miller before, to understand the need to change and improve medicine. I wanted to gain their total commitment. I wanted them all to be productive and innovative, whatever their position.

The communication and dialog about the why began person-to-person, but as we grew into a larger company, I came to another mechanism. I began taking thirty minutes at each quarterly all-employee meeting (AEM) to interview a cancer patient. The patient and I sat in easy chairs recalling their experience discovering their cancer, being diagnosed, and being treated. These candid interactions gave everyone from PhDs to janitors an intimate view of the complexity of cancer diagnosis and the even greater struggle to endure powerful toxic treatments. For the average employee, most in their thirties, this was a hidden world revealed. They were too young to know much of it, and the details we discussed were unknown to them because the discussion between patient and doctor was typically private, behind closed doors.

Importantly, the details coming out of the interviews revealed how Ventana instruments and tests aided diagnosis and informed treatment, which was often a Roche targeted therapy like Herceptin* for HER2 or Rituximab* for CD20-positive lymphoma. The idea was for each employee to connect the dots to understand how their efforts building new tools had helped the patients they were now personally familiar with.

The consequence of this patient exposure at every AEM over many years was that our staff felt empathy. And they felt urgency. They were like Norma—emotionally all in. They understood the impact of their job inventing, making, delivering, and supporting new tools.

After a while, we built on our collective emotional experience to further articulate and codify our *why* into a mission statement: "To improve the lives of all patients afflicted with cancer." That statement was to further intensify our efforts and became another foundation block in our culture.

Beyond the mission statement, we also took the time to establish a common vocabulary. We hired a business consulting group, Partners in Leadership, to take the entire organization through a further articulation of our cultural beliefs. By this means, the employees synthesized our nine cultural beliefs:

Innovate Now.

Think Customer.

Be Bold.

Deliver Quality.

Align to Shine.

Act on Fact.

Speak Up.

Everyone Counts.

Own It.

Each of these tenets had a further defining sentence. For example, for "Own It," it read, "I own our results, refuse to blame others, and embrace challenge." By this process, with a common set of beliefs and a common vocabulary, we became a cohesive group. It helped us achieve unity of effort. And it ensured our culture went beyond me to all. Among the attributes of a strong culture are its transmissibility and sustainability, and by this process we achieved both. The *why* became company wide.

Beyond the why, I was to become heavily involved in the *how*. After all, it is not enough to just dream and aspire; you have to do it and deliver it. This occurred through my involvement as a member of the Ventana board of directors, and a member of the executive team as the chief medical officer, and the chief scientific officer, which gave me everyday proximity to the how. Often my role was to see that the how was informed by the why.

In the why-to-how equation, the medical narrative was critical. One example comes to mind, which was our constant debate over the economics of our business. A case in point was our catalogue of tests that over time grew to more than 300. This large menu of tests was driven by physician demand.

The business issue was the matter of ROI (return on investment) on each test, which could cost millions of dollars to develop and bring to FDA approval. For the tests that were frequently used daily, there was no issue. But for rarely used tests, say a test used once a month, the ROI would never be realized. Why build what will only lose money? On strict economic terms the business was always ready to quash what we called *the orphan tests*. After all, they only lost money.

This is where the medical narrative and the *why* came in. Economics aside, the orphan tests might be rarely used and give no ROI, but they could be critical to patient care. A case in point was the special stain test we sold for detecting Mycobacterium tuberculosis (MTBC). For a comatose patient in the emergency room presenting with tuberculous meningitis, the immediate identification in the MTBC in the cerebral spinal fluid could lead to curative action; without it, disaster. So, a given test in the catalogue might be rarely used, but it might be of vital need.

This then was where I had a constant refrain that we were not just selling tests and instruments; we were selling the high-level practice of medicine for patients' benefit. To hammer this point home, I often made the analogy to selling the alphabet. It went something like this:

If our Ventana sales team, instead of selling tests, was selling letters of the alphabet, our financial team would favor selling vowels (a, e, i, o, u) over the infrequently used consonants (j, q, x, z), since the frequent use of vowels in every word and the rare use of the odd consonants would provide a positive ROI for the vowels and a negative ROI for the consonants. That would be an analytically correct financial finding.

That would only be okay if we were just selling letters, but if we were selling the ability to compose words, write sentences, create paragraphs, and write a whole book, then we needed to sell the whole alphabet.

If our goal was to enable writers to write books, our ROI should be based on the number of books written and sold. And so my constant refrain was we were not just selling tests and instruments, we were selling the practice of medicine and the patient experience. From this refrain came the understanding that we needed to sell the whole catalogue of tests, not just the frequently used ones. It was established that the value of the test was its vital purpose, not the frequency of use. It was this medical narrative, this medical imperative, which was to drive this business for thirty years on.

And so it was that I set the foundation of our culture based on the need to improve medicine. We would do this by providing new tools and new capabilities. I reinforced this medical narrative in every AEM through patient interviews and by being the medical voice in the dollars-and-cents discussions. Finally, as the chief scientific officer, I saw to it that our R & D expenditures were to reflect medical need, not just financial gain.

Cultural aspiration was one thing, but the transmission of that culture to *all* employees was a greater, more arduous challenge. This further articulation of our culture came over the years from our several CEOs, all of whom were strong, smart, energetic, effective leaders whose 24/7 example was instrumental in setting the pace and producing a cohesive team effort.

The one who had the most profound effect was Chris Gleeson. He was our captain and commander for over ten years. He began in 1999, and over his remarkably eventful tenure he led us through thirty-six high-performing quarters on NASDAQ and finally, in 2008, through the negotiation and completion of our acquisition by Roche.

These accomplishments aside, it was Chris, you might say, who was responsible for Norma's tears on that July day in 2003 in NYC.

How so? Because it was Chris who insisted that our moment of glory on NASDAQ would include our star employees of all ranks and positions, not just the top brass. This was representative of Chris's style of leadership by inclusion. He was the one who understood and recognized it was the Normas of the company who were its heart and soul, not just senior leadership. He made every employee a committed contributor and innovator. His methods for creating this dynamic culture were multifarious. He led by example, by constant engagement, inclusion, egalitarianism, and urgency, and by turning difficulty into action, problems into opportunity, blame into accountability, discomfort into comfort, and failure into success. He fit Winston Churchill's prescription for success by overcoming failure after failure with unabated enthusiasm.

When I think back to Chris, he was bristling with unabated enthusiasm. He was fidgeting for action. When I think of his kinetic energy, I think of Teddy Roosevelt driving the building of the Panama Canal. Where others had failed, he prevailed through sheer will. I think of Teddy Roosevelt at San Juan Hill in 1898. Like Teddy, Chris was an instinctive take-the-hill, dodge-the-bullets, defy-the-odds leader. And when you're building new instruments and tests, as we were doing over his ten years, that is the mindset you must have.

Speaking of heroic battles fought, in 1898 Teddy had just one hill. In 2007, Chris had five hills—make that battles—going on at once: (1) the Roche "hostile takeover"; (2) the CytoLogix federal court case; (3) the acquisition of Spring Bioscience; (4) the launch of our second-generation instrument; and the ever-present, never-forget (5) fight to make the quarter's financials for Wall Street, which, if not made, meant we would be acquired for a song. It's one thing to fight a battle, but to face five battles at once and to ultimately win all five was heroic.

As a former Australian military officer, Chris would have relished the comparison to Teddy. He would have relished being called a bull moose. Beyond sharing Teddy's military bearing and daring,

Chris added an air of Aussie-rules football to the daily proceedings, leading us all with an ever-enthusiastic cheer, "AVAGOYERMUG" (literal English translation: "Have a go, you mug," or "Come on, let's go") a traditional rallying call at Aussie-rules football matches. No matter the difficulty, he would end with, "No worries, mate!" An affirmation of his imperturbability. His affability in the face of difficulty was always intact. His comfort with discomfort became a cultural attribute he passed on to us all.

Beyond his leadership by example, Chris was to foster our culture of innovation and egalitarianism by inclusion and engagement.

His engagement with employees was always a priority. It was especially noticeable in his nearly daily walkabouts. On those walks, at the shop and cubicle level, he greeted all by name, and the hands-on workers knew they had status in the CEO's eyes. By the attention he gave to all he encountered, everyone was made to feel important, and their work effort was made visible.

This method of walkabout management, popularized by Hewlett and Packard years ago, sounds like an obvious winner, except in actual practice it often is not. The reason being, in a plant with a thousand people, most encounters last thirty seconds, and the most common topic is the weather. Too many people, too little time. In that limited encounter, employees wanting to impress the boss with their competence would typically speak of some recent success. The real deep-seated problems, the 800-pound gorillas, were not appropriate for a thirty-second interaction. Besides, who wants to be known as a complainer or a whiner?

Chris had a brilliant method to overcome this flaw. First, he took his time. Second, everyone knew he would stay and listen if necessary. The clock be damned, dwelling mattered. Third, he was armed with three magical questions: (1) What's your job? (2) Do you have what you need to do your job? And the most important of all, (3) If you were me, if you were the boss, what would you do to improve the place?

The third question was the magical one. It freed the employee of being labeled a complainer or appearing just self-absorbed. It invited the employee to make the company's progress priority one.

Freedom to become the boss, even for a short time, was a liberating experience. By this means, everyone was made to feel connected, included, and important. By this means, all were invited to improve and create. Once you get a thousand people thinking about the need to improve, the innovations come daily. As I learned before from my graduate students and technicians, give a human being an arduous, repetitive, demanding task, and they quickly imagine a better, more inventive way, which Chris was constantly being schooled in.

Besides his walkabout method of management, Chris brought engagement, inclusiveness, and inventiveness directly to our on-location manufacturing plant by instituting the KEIZAN method, which had been perfected by Toyota in Japan. KEIZAN involved fabricators who were formed into teams and periodically taken off-line to spend a week observing the other production teams. By the end of this week, they were charged with submitting a plan to improve production. Over time, this elevated those individuals from just fabricators, from just *doing* to also *thinking* and creating new or improved processes. They invariably came up with a better way to build. I guess Adam Smith in 1776 was right.

Over time, due to the inclusiveness of all, due to the invitation at the cubicle and shop level to imagine and invent, we were to enjoy a wellspring of patents, altogether an astonishing 900-plus patents over thirty years.

This patent portfolio, representing the keys to the kingdom in a biotech company, was the grand consequence of our intellectual diversity and egalitarianism. Looking back after thirty years at our 900-plus patents issued, many of the names on the patents were employees without an advanced degree. The patent filings often began as records of invention coming from those hands-on employees. Many were patents to manufacturing processes and instrument-refining methods. Altogether, about half of the inventors were engineers and PhD scientists at the university level (e.g., the University of Arizona). Another quarter were lab technicians who had typically graduated from a community college (e.g., Pima College). And another quarter were manufacturing fabricators, often coming from technical schools (e.g., ABC Tech). Chris's engagement and encouragement of the employees from community colleges, technical schools, and those with associate degrees gave us a collective intelligence beyond compare. This became a sterling example of the product of intellectual diversity born from an inclusive boss and an inclusive culture—a creative ecology.

In retrospect, when Chris was walking around, it was not just that he invited employees of every rank into the inner circle of leaders, but rather, in the process of drawing out their inventive ideas, he was being invited into their even larger circle of inventive ideas. As we all learned, the bigger the circle, the stronger the culture.

That was the flavor of the culture born at the shop and cubicle level. Chris used other methods at the level of managers, project leaders, scientists, and engineers. One was born of an ingenious and remarkably effective fifteen-minute project-review process. Here's how it worked:

Two days of every month were dedicated to reviewing the progress of projects. In those two days, twenty projects might be reviewed, and Chris's method was to give each one fifteen minutes. Over time, we all learned the formula—one minute for accomplishments; two minutes for problems; ten minutes for corrective actions, including the call for resources and timelines; and the last two minutes for input from Chris and senior management.

Why just one minute for accomplishments? Because Chris knew

we all had a job building instruments and assays never built before. He knew the rule was daily failure. He knew it was not a tunnel with a light at the end but a maze with frequent dead ends. He knew that gilding the lily about some minor success was just masking the true difficulty. He didn't like the guise of self-accomplishment hiding the problems, the dead ends. Thus, the good news was always cut short. And if you were so brazen as to brag on and on, then you risked being seen as a "poppy too tall," which is Australian disdain for a person posing and bragging to outshine others. The poppy too tall invariably brought out Chris's wrath and made him "mad as a frilled lizard," as they sometimes are Down Under.

Why just two minutes for bad news? Don't complicated problems require extended analysis? As Chris saw it, extended analysis fostered paralysis. He favored solving problems by taking action. He had a host of Aussie-isms to express his no-nonsense approach.

"Just spit out the problem, mate."

"Tell it as it is, even if it's a dog's breakfast."

No *coulda, woulda, shoulda* excuses. Don't blame circumstance or others, just get to the solution, the action, the urgency. He didn't want you devoting your brain power to floundering. Turn it into action.

Why ten minutes for corrective actions? Because over time it taught us to devote most of our brain power to solutions. He wanted every problem connected to an action plan. He would say, "Give me the four or five possible actions, including how many people, to what end, in what time frame. Tell me what we don't know and how we will learn more."

Absorbed as we all became in the action plan, we learned by this means that every problem presented an opportunity. He gave us an optimist's view of difficulty. He taught us how an optimist with a plan is happy to be discomforted by a problem because it's an opportunity to learn. Over time, we became comfortable with being discomforted. Ultimately over many years of this optimistic formula, taking problems by the horns, we were only truly discomforted if things appeared too comfortable. We favored diligence and feared laxity. Letting a problem lie was the worst.

Why the last two minutes for Chris? In those two minutes Chris, as the CEO, drew his conclusions and decided which plan, which resources, which timeline. There was no delayed analysis, no committee to defer to. No paralysis by further analysis. Just judgment and conclusion.

The boss, by God, had decided. There was buy-in at the top. The body and the head were connected. The nervous system was connected to the musculoskeletal system. The whole body could now move into action.

In the last minute, when the boss, hearing all the facts and action plans, gave his guidance (do this, not that; do it by then; do it with these resources), he was creating a contract. He was sharing the logic, setting expectations, and he was also crossing the boundary from blame to accountability.

The distinction between blame and accountability was critical to Chris and all those around him. To the one assigned the task, failure was always possible, but if you acted according to plan with full effort, then failure may be judged regrettable but not blameworthy. If you had done your job, failure was not because of you. Blame was not in the equation. Given the employee's full effort, failure was not personalized. It was not taken as a personal defeat (the ultimate demoralizer). Failure is shared. Failure in this instance taught us all we were united in our temporary defeat. Our understanding and comfort with failure ultimately allowed us to overcome our collective ignorance. It motivated us to find new knowledge acquired by failure, which is among the most precious types of knowledge. Our acquired comfort with failure, our lack of blame with full effort, allowed us to fulfill Churchill's prescription for success by enduring failure with unabated enthusiasm.

Our shared failure and the valuable knowledge we gained from it came to be seen as a strength, a virtue, not a weakness. A culture is especially strong when it carries you through the troughs to the high ground.

Beyond his walk-around and meeting-engagement practices, Chris imposed a third method to ensure intellectual diversity—succession planning. At his insistence, all managers presenting their five to six yearly major business objectives (MBOs) were to have at least one that outlined their plan to ensure members of their team were being schooled and groomed to replace the manager over time. That provision meant a manager's success and bonuses required documenting that they had uplifted members of their team. This provision turned all the leaders into mentors, which over the years ensured a steady stream of well-trained individuals fit for promotion. By this means, glass ceilings in management were shattered by design.

This constant schooling of the company managers by Chris had a strong positive effect within the company, but it also raised and motivated a whole generation of future leaders. As it turns out, eight of them were to spread their wings and become CEOs of other biotech companies. Once again, our considerable effort to ensure genuine successors gave our culture transmissibility to the next generation, ensuring sustainability and future company success.

Finally, the abiding consequence of our well-established culture was a sustained record of invention. From the original IHC/ISH instruments and a handful of tests, we were to build a second- and then third-generation instrument. We also broadened our scope to develop an automated H&E stainer, a special stainer for infectious agents, and an image analyzer, and our catalogue grew to more than 300 assays. The common denominator in all that technological growth was a strong culture fostering motivation and innovation.

After all this serious cultural-growth talk, Mom nodded approvingly. She loved hearing of Norma again. She knew Chris well, and all the talk of him spurred her to remember a favorite story I used to tell about Chris and how he would revert to Aussie speak. It was a recollection of a voicemail message from Chris Gleeson to me delivered on August 20, 2000, at 2:30 a.m. He was agitated about a project gone south and about a manager under my supervision who failed to give full effort. As I have explained, full effort generally left one blameless, but on the other hand, if you failed to show full effort, if you failed to follow plan, and if you failed to communicate, then you were accountable and bore personal responsibility for the failure, and you would likely be fired.

Anyway, without the decorum of a formal meeting, just between us in private he let fly, and as he often did when mad, he reverted to Aussie speak.

"Tom, I am mad as a frilled lizard. The whole project looks like a dog's breakfast. The thing has Buckley's chance for success, and you told me it was a piece of piss. Come on, the bloke you put in charge is a bloody dingo up a gum tree. He's running around like a headless chook. I sticky beaked this, and I am ready to stir the possum. All I can say about your management style, mate, is you're like a cocky on a biscuit tin and nothing but a bogan. That's all for now. We'll talk tomorrow. No worries, mate."

Fortunately, by that time I had acquired an Australian-English dictionary and set to the translation. I realized it was not an endorsement of my own management style and left me realizing I needed to stir the possum, too!

13.

Family Matters

WHEN MARTIN DEMPSEY WAS CHAIRMAN of the Joint Chiefs of Staff and head of the US military he said, "When a soldier goes to war, so does the spouse." To put it another way, when I went on my quest, so did my wife and family. If a man chooses to climb Mount Everest, so does his wife, even if she is just following along at home with the kids. In my case, my wife, Cande, and kids, Emily and Andrew, adapted to my quest with one of their own. And as it turned out, I can say I never would have succeeded in the medical instrument business if my wife and kids had not succeeded in the restaurant business.

As Dempsey knew from multiple tours in Afghanistan and Iraq, it takes a supportive, happy family to keep a soldier happy, and to keep him fighting. In a family, you are only as happy as your least happy member. A spouse's inattention to wife or husband, or a father or mother's inattention to daughter or son, could understandably spawn discord and unhappiness. At some point, inattention can leave a child emotionally orphaned. The Everest climber may find satisfaction upon reaching the top, but what satisfaction do the ones at home get? If you have your own ambition, why must it be subservient to another's?

When my father was being helicoptered into Mogadishu, why would my mom, stuck with three kids in Cyprus, feel fulfilled? The fact is they both had a job to do. Dad with the bad guys, and Mom with her brood of unschooled boys. They both succeeded because they had achieved General Dempsey's ideal of "clarity of purpose and unity of effort."[8] They had high purpose and high commitment and a cohesive unit, which—as any Navy 6 SEAL unit proves—is a powerful thing.

When the mob in Nicosia set out to burn the British library under the revolutionary banner of ENOSIS in 1954, when they spotted our British car and headed straight for us like killer bees, it was Mom who jumped into action, hit the accelerator, and plowed through. Sometimes a supportive role involves a lot more than waiting. Sometimes support staff must fight too. My success took patience and perseverance, and Cande was the bedrock for both pillars.

Cande was brought up as the daughter of a Navy chaplain, a Presbyterian minister. She was accustomed to frequent moves and the challenge of new and different circumstances. She was taught not to complain or wither waiting, but to support, encourage, and endure. She accepted my twelve years of working two jobs and losing money. We sometimes felt a slave to unreasonable, unobtainable aspirations. High purpose can be a tyrant, and lost time and lack of economic gain are tyrants that can haunt and exhaust.

Cande did not surrender. She knew passivity was not the answer. She didn't just watch me climb. She climbed her own mountain. In fact, she was to climb two mountains—one she chose, and one that chose her.

First, the mountain she chose. It was to be a tough, arduous climb that led her to become the owner and proprietor of a first-rate Tucson restaurant known as Ovens.

Her story began forty years ago, after ten years of marriage, when we moved to Palo Alto, where I started a fellowship in hematopathology at Stanford. After we moved in, Cande began restlessly looking to expand her horizons, as both our children, Emily and Andrew, were in school all day. The search was brief. She was drawn to an ad in *The Stanford Daily* by a Stanford professor soliciting a private chef. Besides being a famous professor of psychology, he had a startup, and between the two he was constantly entertaining. He had grown tired of going to the same old restaurants and decided to switch to entertaining at his on-campus home. He wanted a private chef who knew both classic and modern *cuisine minceur* French cuisine. Cande, after interviewing, became that chef. The combination of her prior six-year experience in San Francisco cooking schools and her winning personality got her the job. And so, over the next year she launched her newfound career, which ended in her co-owning two restaurants in Tucson.

The Palo Alto experience proved highly formative for her. The professor had a marvelous idiosyncrasy; he didn't want the same dish twice—unless, of course, he loved it. But the call for endless variety was to become Cande's graduate school in cuisine. As any graduate student seeking intellectual gain will tell you, the demands of a great professor are the path, however demanding, to new knowledge. In that year, Cande found her inner Julia Child. At least twice a week for a year, she began her preparation in our home kitchen.

The memories of the glorious smells and tastes of her culinary concoctions still linger. As I came through the door at the end of the hospital workday, she was packing baskets with savories and sweets. The waft of just-baked *madeleines*, just-braised *coq au vin* and just-frosted *dacquoise-au-chocolat* was enough to have driven Marcel Proust to tears. Her lobster Plaza Athénée, to be served before her saddle of lamb *en croute* followed by her *gateau marjolaine*, would have made Jacques Pépin weep openly. Her *foie gras en croute* was Fernand Point worthy, and her *tarte Tatin* was Gaston Lenôtre worthy. All this sensory phantasmagoria was a-swirl in the just-exited kitchen as she packed up and left for the professor's house with her moveable

Babette's feast. Our Louisa Trotter of London culinary fame was off to regale royalty (upstairs) while the kids and I settled in at the kitchen table (downstairs) to tuck away our mac and cheese.

Cande's culinary graduate school days, while glorious and triumphant, were to end when I took a position as an assistant professor at the University of Arizona. As she was fully aware, we were moving to the edge of the known universe, and the odds were against finding a culinary patron like the Stanford professor. In the land of hot chiles and pinto beans, the call for lobster Athénée or *dacquoise-au-chocolat* was unlikely. But, as all great cooks and military kids do, she adapted to circumstance and geography. As Julia taught her, if the soufflé falls, cover it with raspberry sauce and call it a pudding. It didn't take long for Cande to transition from *beef bourguignon* to stuffed poblano chiles, from *gateau marjolaine* to Mexican *tres leches* cakes. She adapted quickly to the new ingredients, but the career path was less certain and, unquestionably, opportunities were fewer. In the face of uncertainty, childrearing and husband-supporting, her career went into dormancy.

As time passed, and the children grew more independent, and the husband more preoccupied on his seven-million-mile quest, Cande, now Southwest-adapted, was ready for new prospects. It began again as catering from home, but there was greater ambition. She quickly joined with two partners to start a combined catering and cooking-school business and commenced to raise the culinary bar at the edge of the known universe. That successful enterprise led to starting a Southwest-cuisine restaurant, Café Terra Cotta, which became an overnight success, including national coverage in the *New York Times* and on PBS. The restaurant was a triumph. Cande was born again as a restaurateur. The success was sweet, but there was to be a parting of ways with her partners. Undaunted, Cande, with a new partner, Jim Caljean, started a unique new bistro known as Ovens, where she again found culinary success, this time with a fusion of Southwest and French/Italian cuisine.

Her success coincided with my sustained difficulties at Ventana. After a decade, Ventana was still down $50 million, and I was still on an academic's salary, barely scraping by. But Cande's consistent profit as a restaurateur kept the family afloat. Her wood-fired poblano pizzas, roasted chicken with garlic mashed potatoes, and her always-beloved *tarte Tatin* kept the whole family on terra firma.

After the day job at the U, and a few hours at the V, I was off to eat at the O, where my wife presided, my daughter, Emily, hosted, and my son, Andrew, bussed. I had the nightly reassurance that my own uncommon, demanding quest was met by their equally uncommon adaptation to their own quests. We had achieved Dempsey's clarity of purpose and unity of effort.

It was at this moment Cande declared we as a couple could now be said to have defined a new marriage paradigm—the bi-entrepreneurial couple! Perhaps something Neil Simon could write a play about, although at this point we did not know whether the play should be a comedy or a tragedy. Do you go with Elaine May and Mike Nichols or Elizabeth Taylor and Richard Burton? Given the level of stress, it could, after all, end as Edward Albee's *Who's Afraid of Virginia Woolf.* But then again, that's the thing about becoming bi-entrepreneurial; it's a state of mutual respect and admiration that Albee's characters lacked.

It was at the height of this newly found unity of effort that our fortune changed. It was August of 2005 when misfortune struck in the form of cancer. As it turned out, Cande was to climb a second mountain. This was not the one she chose; it was the one that chose her. It happened like this:

On a Friday morning in mid-August 2005, after a rich restaurant meal the night before, Cande had a bout of abdominal pain, nausea, and vomiting. The severity led her to the university medical center a few blocks away, where a sonogram was done, suspecting gallstones common in middle-aged, multiparous women. The surprise was finding a peach-sized mass in the retroperitoneum near the ureter. A CT-scan biopsy was to follow, but the intravenous iodine-based dye produced an immediate dramatic allergic reaction, requiring high-dose steroids. She was then given an alternative non-iodine contrast medium.

The next challenge was to determine the nature of the beast. Was it benign or malignant? As the attending, awaiting diagnostician, I was hopeful of benignancy. Cande's long-standing migraine headaches had been treated with ergot-based drugs, which could cause a benign fibrosis in the retroperitoneum. Alas, the biopsy under the microscope was unequivocally malignant. The tumor had the single-cell appearance of a lymphoma, but the primitive, anaplastic cells looked like an immature leukemia.

It was undeniably a lethal threat, and the odds of incurability were overwhelming. Given all the commotion and tension of the past two days, I made the decision not to awaken Cande, and not to speak to her that evening of the lethality and incurability. I would let her rest, and on Sunday would confer and confront the further difficulty.

That night, as I went home to sleep, I felt an impending sense of doom. How to put it? How to speak and comfort when you feel dread? My answer was, before bed, to call Dr. Miller. As my longstanding colleague and friend, Tom was the man we needed, she needed, I needed. He was the oncologist who would be able to explain the fight ahead, to lead and guide us through. After we spoke on the phone, we agreed to meet at seven in the morning, and to proceed together to bring the news to Cande.

Before that meeting with Dr. Miller, there was a surprise. Unprompted by me, my techs, Catherine and Yvette Fruitiger, had pulled an all-nighter. Reading my stress, they spent all night rendering the chemistry on Cande's biopsy. Looking to determine the nature of the beast, they ran more than thirty IHC assays on a Ventana instrument and enticed our fellow, Marina Jaramillo, to stay up with them and read the slides. By 6 a.m., Marina called me saying there was a major surprise, and I should come to the lab ASAP to see.

Over the phone, Marina said the surprise was that, despite the primitive appearance of the tumor, it was in fact a CD20-positive large B-cell lymphoma known to be one of the most curable of all cancers.

I immediately called Dr. Miller and picked him up early at his home. As we drove to the hospital lab, I questioned, how could this be? What explained the discrepancy between the frightening cells I saw microscopically and the more reassuring chemistry? Considering the perplexity, Dr. Miller—ever the medical Sherlock Holmes—surmised the answer.

"Steroid . . . *steroids*, that's it!" he blurted. "It's the steroids given on Friday because of her allergic reaction that acted on the tumor and gave the cells the scary blastic appearance." He went on. The steroids, well known to affect lymphocytes, had changed the appearance of the malignant lymphocytes and thereby tricked us at the microscope, but the tissue chemistry saved the day by giving us the true nature of the beast.

Dr. Miller became further animated. "This is the critter I know. This is the critter we can cure. Let's go after it—let's start right now!"

The team at the lab was also excited. Catherine, Yvette, and Marina stood by the tray of IHC slides like an obstetrical team that had just delivered a baby. A baby indeed. As the slides showed, it was undeniably a CD20-positive diffuse large B-cell lymphoma.

Without hesitation, the team was off to Cande's hospital room. Before all, Dr. Miller gave her the news. He explained the large-cell lymphoma was a lethal threat, but that, as proven by Catherine, Yvette, and Marina, it was a CD20-positive large B-cell type for which there was a highly efficacious targeted anti-CD20 therapy, Rituximab*, available from Genentech/Roche. The Rituximab* coupled with standard chemotherapy (CHOP) had a high probability of cure, if given monthly for eight months. In an instant, the lethal threat turned into a strong prospect for cure.

After scans the next day, Cande was given Rituximab* plus chemo intravenously. After the first infusion, Dr. Miller came calling, emphasizing the treatment likely killed 99 percent of the tumor. The next eight months' treatments were designed to get the last tumor cell, to chase the last invisible threat.

In those ninety-six hours, Cande had gone from seeming robust health, to a lethal threat, to a highly informed diagnosis, to a well-articulated target of therapy, to the infusion of curative-intent therapy. As vexing and unexpected as it all was to Cande, her support team was ecstatic. To them, her diagnosis and treatment was a triumph of technology between the CT-guided biopsy, the automated overnight IHC, and the targeted therapy. To them, it was the harmonic convergence of radiology, pathology, chemistry, oncology, and pharmacology.

It was having the right tools at the right time to find the beast, characterize the beast, and treat the beast, knowing its vulnerabilities. These were high-quality results delivered quickly at the place Cande lived, at the time she needed it, to receive immediate therapy without prolonged anxiety. We all agreed, this was the experience all patients—not just doctors' wives—should have in every hospital, in every city, in every country of the world. This was to become the goal for Ventana and Roche Tissue Diagnostics over the next fifteen years, realized first by Cande.

Of all the stories I told, this one was Mom's favorite because she reveled in Cande's assertive steadfast adaptation to the difficulties thrown her way. She especially admired Cande's resolve and courage in the face of a life-threatening illness. Mom also admired Cande's ability to adapt to her husband's uncommon choices, as she had done herself in the Middle East and Africa. And she liked that Emily and Andrew adapted and found their own purpose and direction.

As pleased as she was with the recollection, she was quick to correct me regarding the bi-entrepreneurial family, pointing out that I should call it quad-entrepreneurial, as both Emily and Andrew had founded and run their own private businesses.

Emily, having hosted and waitressed for her mom, went on to a nearly twenty-year career as a stage actress, starting as Juliet in *Romeo and Juliet* and ending as Anna in *Anna Karenina*. Then, retiring from acting and reschooling, she emerged as a psychology counselor in her own private practice. She switched from playing the likes of a Chekov character to counseling them in her office. Emily's high social intelligence followed her from restaurateur to acting to counseling.

Andrew was to establish his own geospatial information company, having spent over a decade doing what is called tactical urban spatial geography—basically making three-dimensional electronic maps of places like Fallujah during the Iraq war and Abbottabad in pursuit of the likes of Osama Bin Laden. After all, flying a helicopter at night at a ground-hugging altitude with multiple rendezvous sites requires precise three-dimensional maps drawn from satellite telemetry.

Amazingly, thirty years after his grandfather's time, Andrew— like his grandfather before him—was to become preoccupied with chasing bad guys, whether the Taliban, Bin Laden, or Isis. His inclination might be congenital, coming from his grandfather's side.

14.

Perry Mason Moment

MOM RARELY ASKED FOR LEGAL details of my business. She found them too contentious and unsettling. But there was one major case she wanted me to recall. I think because it took place in federal court in Boston, near my parents' home in Exeter, New Hampshire, just forty miles away. I think what she liked about the case was that for a month, I had been home on the weekends. And Dad and I were then sometimes off to the salt marsh in Seabrook to drift a fly for sea-run striped bass. Also, my two brothers were often there. My brother Buzz, back from his startup company in Taiwan, and Tim, my mentally disabled brother, were also home for the weekend. So, as rarely happened, to her great pleasure, the family was intact.

Once a new product is established and a company becomes profitable, and its success is visible on Wall Street, the added public attention has consequences—some good, some vexing. Among the good, the growing financial strength attracts even more capital; bees are drawn to the honey. Customers also observe the public strength and sign up for longer-term contracts, knowing the company is stable, no longer a scrape-by startup. At the same time, competitors are also drawn to the honey. This too can be a positive as the involvement of multiple companies reassures investors of sector strength, and customers of possible alternative choices.

More vexing is the competition. As other companies try to piggy-back on your inventions, it turns contentious and legal over critical matters of intellectual property (IP). After all, the business is predicated on game-changing, patent-protected inventions. Patents codify and formalize the IP so it can be put to public use and, if necessary, defended in court.

Patents, because they endure a rigorous, critical independent scientific review at the patent office, help to validate the foundation of a business. They ensure the freedom to operate that is so critical to a technology-driven company. The most effective way to build a strong foundation in a new technical company is to go beyond the first patent to establish a patent portfolio by continuing to invent and continuing to improve the product. The patents then come to define and protect the instruments and tests you've invented. Even more protection is gained by patenting the means and materials for manufacture. Following this approach for over thirty years, our patent portfolio grew to more than 900 globally.

As impregnable as 900 patents may seem to legal assault, gaps always remain. The best way to think of a patent portfolio is by analogy to a picket fence. To have a fully functional fence, you need to have all the pickets in place. Even though we aggressively gave high priority to continuous inventions, we were still missing a few pickets.

So, like General Motors having all the patents it requires for the engine but needing one for an intermittent windshield wiper, the needed IP must be licensed, bought, or legally contested. Over the years, some ten or twelve times, we either bought or licensed our needed pickets.

On several occasions, after considerable saber rattling and legal threats, we concluded a negotiation by trading pickets on the principle that it was better for both parties to have freedom to operate; better to spend the money on their customers and not waste it on drawn-out legal battles. The most commonly bartered IP licenses occurred with larger medical diagnostic companies. On rare occasions, it came to proceedings in federal court, some of which we won, and some we lost. But in the end, all were settled legally and financially to ensure our ongoing freedom to operate.

One of our most contentious legal battles was fought in August 2007 in a federal court in Boston. Ventana, by then growing by leaps and bounds, was accused of monopolistic practices by a Boston startup company that had briefly competed with automation but failed. Specifically, the accusation was that we had illegally and unjustly dominated them. We were further accused of using our position of strength—having most of the automated-instrument market—to undercut them by manipulating price, rushing new features to market, and overwhelming customers by badmouthing the newbie.

There was a substantial body of antitrust law going back to the Gilded Age and the robber barons that forbade monopolistic practices. History taught that laissez-faire capitalism required legal limitations.

After seven years of depositions and legal wrangling, we found ourselves before a jury and a federal judge of the Fifth Circuit Court of Appeals. It was a high-stakes, bet-the-company trial, accusing us of monopolistic practices and threatening triple damages in the range of $300 million.

As we walked to the court from the hotel that first morning to begin jury selection, our legal team buzzed with anticipation. They were ready to fight, and I was feeling nauseated.

Our legal warriors from Kirkland & Ellis of Chicago were first-rate. They were confident in their legal arguments, but they had one major concern—me.

I was there as the face of the defense—the human face the jury would associate with our adversary's accusations of nefarious behavior. I was to be portrayed by the other side as the robber baron of old who had crushed a hard-working, well-intended group of Bostonians. As an experienced litigator, our Kirkland attorney, Mike Fordas, understood that an emotionally unstable defendant could unfavorably distract the attention of the jury away from the legal facts and get them fixated on the alleged treachery of the accused. So, as we walked to legal Armageddon, leather on concrete, on the sidewalk by the Boston South station, he stopped me.

"Okay, Tom," Fordas said. "What's happening here?"

"I think I may throw up," I responded.

"What's the problem?" he pressed.

"Oh, I don't know," I shot back. "Just the threat of a $300-million judgment against us that could obliterate twenty years of effort. Just the demise of a company employing a thousand people. Just the end of all we've built."

"Tom," Fordas urged. "No, no, no! Stop. Don't do this. Don't worry. We have good arguments."

"Mike," I replied. "For you they're arguments. For me and a thousand others, it's a lifetime down the drain."

"Look," he said. "The facts are on our side. The jury will hear us. We will win."

"Your faith in the jury astounds me," I replied.

"Why? Your peers will understand," he assured me.

"Really?" I insisted. "We are the carpet-baggers here. We are appearing before a jury of Bostonians. It will be unequivocal home cooking. And to top it off, the jury we are about to select will be composed of the night shift from McDonald's. They will naturally favor the failed, seek to punish the successful, and enjoy the chance to take a shot at the robber baron, the capitalist pig!"

"Settle down," Fordas replied. "I disagree. In fact, I'd rather try this case in Boston, in front of a Boston jury, than in your hometown of Tucson, Arizona!"

"What, are you nuts?" I was incredulous. "Why?"

"Because," he responded, "our defense is factual, technical, detailed, and analytical. And, as you're about to witness, we have a better chance at a PhD or engineer on the jury in Boston than in Arizona. And that's all I need—just one technologically knowledgeable person."

As it turned out, Fordas was right. Even as the plaintiff sought to strike every technologically savvy prospective juror, we ended up with two PhDs and a medical device engineer. And in the end, it was the medical device–savvy engineer who gave us the dramatic Perry Mason moment that won the day.

That moment came ten days into a three-week trial, in which we were accused of monopolistic behavior. As the face of the defense, as the accused robber baron, I sat at the defense table facing the jury, the judge, and the witnesses.

The plaintiff's attorney had relentlessly presented our "monopolistic" misbehaviors. The jury was shown our sales materials touting our anthem, "Crush them like a bug." They saw the Tom-and-Jerry cartoon in our sales materials that showed Tom (us) swallowing Jerry (them) whole. Etcetera, etcetera, etcetera. All of this presented as evidence of our dominating behavior. More seriously, they accused us of secretly obtaining their business plan, of selling our products at a loss and, finally, of rushing a new instrument to market to trump them.

After ten days, the situation felt like Napoleonic law, in which the accused is guilty until proven innocent. The jury seemed ready to go to judgment, ready to punish the robber baron.

Though I was coached by my legal team to remain cool and collected, my emotions were hard to check. I took being judged a greedy, bullying capitalist pig as painfully unfair. Didn't they understand where I started? The sacrifices that were made? I came from a working-class family; my parents had sacrificed every penny for my schooling. My dad, late in his career, turned down a plush London assignment to take risky duty in Africa in exchange for extra combat pay to ensure my medical school and my brother Buzz's engineering school costs were covered. Didn't they realize my own twenty-year effort with Ventana had not yet achieved my vision? Yes, I had stock options and may have seemed the fat cat, but those were likely worthless given the legal threat before us. These strong feelings, though, were legally irrelevant, so I did my best to keep my emotions in check.

Although I knew the accusations were overblown and unfair, I avoided eye contact, avoided being emotional, and sat methodically filling in a notebook focused on the factual. By the time I had recorded the umpteenth misdeed, and the tide of accusations was at its highest, the ebb came at last.

It came unexpectedly as a sudden surge.

The professor of monopoly law had just completed his third hour of testifying, having listed and detailed thirty-eight violations. The federal judge had just dismissed him. He had risen in the witness box and had one foot in the air when across the room a juror raised his hand. The professor paused. The judge inquired. The juror spoke. "Your honor, may the jury ask questions?"

"Of course you may," the judge replied. "Professor, sit down, please."

"Professor," the juror said. "Would you answer the question? Is the product the automated instrument, or is the product the microscopic slide assay?"

The professor considered for a moment and then answered, "The microscopic slide assay."

"Thank you," said the juror.

"Is that all?" the judge asked.

"Yes, your honor," the juror confirmed.

That question and the professor's four-word answer revealed all. This was the Perry Mason moment, as in the singular dramatic event that changed the whole proceeding. How could four words change everything? What was the legal significance? How would a juror, as a layperson, know the legal crux of the matter?

Through his question, the juror showed a critical understanding of the guiding principle of antitrust law, that the all-knowing, learned law professor had slyly not mentioned. As the juror quite amazingly comprehended, that principle was *control*. That is, in order to dominate and misbehave in a monopolistic way, you must be in control of a market, as AT&T and Ma Bell once were, or as the robber barons were with steel (Carnegie), oil (Rockefeller), and the railroad (Vanderbilt) monopolies.

In his account of the thirty-eight misdeeds, the professor had amply cited voluminous legal case history. His case comparisons, as I wrote them down, seemed compelling. But as he delved into many written volumes of relevant case law, it turned out that he had skipped over the first paragraph of volume number one. He had jumped right to *Revelations* without covering *Genesis.* Instead of starting, "In the beginning," he went straight to "hellfire and damnation."

Had he read to the jury from the beginning, he would have read that to be a monopolist, you must control a market, meaning that you must have a dominant market share comprising greater than 80 percent.

While it was true that, at the time, relevant to the accusations, we were number one in automated instrument sales, we, nonetheless, did not have control and could not dominate the market. We lacked control because the assays on a glass slide could be performed manually. Indeed, anyone with the reagents, a pipette, and an opposable thumb could do these assays. In fact, at the time in question, the manual, by-hand method was dominant!

So if the product was the automated instrument, we could be said to be dominant and in control, but if the product was the test on the glass slide, then the by-hand method was dominant and in control. By this logic, the thirty-eight accusations were not applicable, and— most amazingly of all—the questioning juror somehow perceived this correctly. Astoundingly, this juror had snatched out of the unspoken words of the professor the crux of the matter. He had correctly perceived the very argument we were planning to make, the "toothbrush argument," which went something like this:

If you were the number one manufacturer of electric toothbrushes and a new competitor entered the market, you could get animated and speak of dominance, of crushing bugs, of devouring the little mouse as we did. This may be rude and uncivil, but it is not monopolistic. Why? Because any customer with a toothbrush and a hand with an opposable thumb can brush their teeth without an electrical device. Indeed, we all know this, since most of us brush our teeth manually. We, the collective manual tooth-brushers, being the vast majority, in fact dominate and, you could say, control the market because the product is the toothbrush, not the new-fangled electric contrivance. Ergo, the toothbrush market never makes it out of the first paragraph of the monopoly law book—and so it was for us, too.

In our case, any lab technician with reagents, a pipette, an opposable thumb, and a glass slide with tissue could manually deliver a result, as Catherine did all those years before, unfettered by automated devices and their manufacturers. So, as with the toothbrush market, the IHC market—at that time dominated by the manual method—did not make it out of the first paragraph of monopolistic law. There may have been uncivil, rude, and even nasty competitive behavior, but not monopolistic.

But how could a lay juror figure this out? How does a lay juror know what a law professor has not presented? There were no lawyers on the jury, so how was this insight possible? As it turned out, the juror with the question, the one with the knowledge and insight, was not strictly speaking a *lay* juror. This was the juror with experience in the medical device industry, a technically knowledgeable engineer. He was a professional aware of the industry and aware of the rules of the game. He knew from experience the rules of fair and unfair competition. Our case was not being judged by the night shift from McDonald's; it was being judged by a true peer as the jury system meant it to be.

The Perry Mason moment had profound consequences. First, our legal team was bolstered and now even more confident in the arguments to follow, so they were steady at the helm. Second, outside the courtroom, events were more dramatic. The outside talks, which commonly occur in business disputes fearing uncertain jury decision, had come to a near agreement of a $100 million settlement. This seemed rational on our side, given the uncertainty and risk at hand.

However, after the eureka moment, our CEO, Chris Gleeson, was convinced we could prevail on a jury judgment, and after a midnight telephone meeting our board of directors, including myself, agreed that the risk of jury verdict was reasonable. Some two weeks later, after our side presented and I got my chance in the witness box, I stood before the jury demonstrating the instrument and the microscopic slide. After I presented the glass slide as the product, the jury went to deliberations and in two hours returned a judgment upholding our defense.

Fordas was right. Finding a knowledgeable group of peers who could adjudicate based on fact, principle, and experience was pivotal. In the end, it was not home cooking. It was not the Red Sox versus the Yankees. It was an understanding of science, technology, and legal principles that prevailed.

There was one final unexpected consequence that Perry Mason, the crack TV lawyer, might have appreciated. It was the day after jury judgment, and it was time to celebrate. One of our defense team lawyers, Jeff Danis, the inventor of the toothbrush defense, was a dyed-in-the-wool Red Sox fan, and so was I, having grown up listening to the Sox on the radio with my grandfather at the lake cabin in New Hampshire. Jeff and I decided that going to a game at Fenway was our reward. The game with the Angels that afternoon was sold out, but after paying $450 to a scalper, we ended up in prime seats behind third base in the sun at field level.

The game was an exhilarating antidote to three weeks of wrangling in court. Beer in plastic cups had a miraculous absolving effect. Baseball talk replaced legal mutterings. Life was good again. There was only one negative. After we were pretty well into our cups, after the banter had become all-absorbing, I alarmed Jeff with a sudden revelation.

"Jeff," I said. "We have a serious problem."

"What problem?" He was confused. "We won. What are you worried about now?"

"Look up," I replied. "Look around. Notice anything?"

"Not really," he said.

"You must be blind," I insisted. "Can't you see we're the only two here?"

"The only two at Fenway?" he asked.

"Yeah," I responded. "I guess the game finished a long time ago. Shouldn't we leave?"

Jeff smiled. "Nah, let's stay. I'll take Fenway over federal court any day."

15.

Becoming Swiss

MOST STARTUPS HAVE A MIND to being acquired. After the IPO, it's the next major payday for the inventors and investors.

Not us. We were on a roll. We were finding new customers, expanding from North America to the EU and Japan. Our revenue was growing by leaps and bounds to double digits. Wall Street analysts liked our mathematics as the growth was sustained and we had turned profitable. They were pleased with their bet on Seabiscuit.

Then came Roche, the fifty-billion-dollar-per-annum Swiss pharmaceutical company that had a long history in diagnostics and a major division devoted to it. Roche was *the* pioneer in the field of precision, or personalized, medicine, which works through a combination of diagnostic tests that determine the characteristics of a patient's disease and smart drugs specifically tailored to be effective in those particular molecular circumstances.

Roche had an eye toward marrying their therapeutics to our automated diagnostics. Through their US biotech unit, Genentech, they already had two blockbuster anti-cancer drugs, an anti-CD20 drug, Rituximab˚, and an anti-HER2 drug, Herceptin˚. Roche's two top executives, Franz Humer, the chairman, and Severin Schwan, the CEO, saw the wisdom of basing the treatment on a proven diagnostic target. In particular, HER2 testing by hand proved problematic in the field; it had an estimated error rate of 20 percent! Consequently, our automation of both the protein and gene tests was attractive to them.

Severin came calling in February 2007. Arriving at the plant in Tucson, he had the bearing and executive presence befitting a CEO of a major global company. He was the model of Swiss propriety and correctness. His manner was polite and proper, but not stiff. The surprise was his genuinely inquisitive manner. It was "Please explain this," or "Tell me more about that," or "Show me more," and "Help me understand." He was all ears.

Curious by nature, Severin came seeking more than the terms of the business deal. He came seeking understanding. He spoke of people in need in distant lands, and not of profit for profit's sake. We shared the view that medicine should be the same everywhere. Whether a deal was struck or not, I felt at that moment the presence of a kindred spirit. And, as I later learned, in an acquisition a kindred spirit helps mightily.

Weeks later, Roche extended a friendly offer of $60 a share for 51 percent of Ventana. It was a generous offer, given that our shares on NASDAQ were then trading near $40. Although the premium of nearly 50 percent over our stock price was attention-getting, the 51-percent ownership was not. At 51 percent, any business downturn meant Roche could buy the remaining 49 percent for a song. Our board of directors quickly united over a loss of control issue and formally rejected the offer. Our chairman, Jack Schuler, said it was our fiduciary responsibility to the shareholders to seek other offers. He invoked our schoolteacher in Wisconsin and her pension fund. He reminded us it was our fiduciary responsibility to seek the maximum value for her.

And so, we held firm, until the surprise of June 26, 2007, when the offer turned hostile. With a $75 share offer, Roche went directly to the shareholders. Suddenly, the Wisconsin schoolteacher's pension fund and all VMSI shareholders had the potential to override our board. It was deemed hostile because it was contrary to the board's unified position. But was it hostile to the Wisconsin fund and all the other NASDAQ institutional and individual investors? Not necessarily. After all, they would receive $75 for a $40 stock. Why not? Well, what if that $40 share was on a growth trajectory to be worth three times as much? Why would you sell a $120 share for $75?

In February 2008, after an eight-month hostile-takeover fight, after innumerable public and private exchanges, after all the wrangling, after our lament of being taken by pirates, we voted, in the name of our fiduciary responsibility, to be taken. We accepted the Swiss tender, realizing $89.50 a share, amounting to a $3.4-billion offer. The shareholders were quick to vote to accept. Fiduciary responsibility realized. By any measure, it was a substantial economic outcome for an idea once rejected thirty-five times.

And so the deal was done, signed, sealed, and delivered. After all the public folderol, I had a sudden private moment alone with the Roche chairman Franz Humer and CEO Severin Schwan. They'd both just arrived from Basel, Switzerland, to address the Ventana employees. Alone with them, knowing they paid a pretty penny, knowing they had found frustration in the public clamor of it all, I felt compelled to ask a simple question. Why? Why go through the bother? Why spend the money? Why take the risk?

Their response? "We need the automated instrument with its capacity to standardize and universalize testing, to ensure our drugs are going to the right patients. We believe this will greatly assist targeted therapy for cancer and help create personalized medicine globally."

Knowing of the many difficulties of manual, by-hand testing, especially of difficult tests like HER2, I understood and appreciated Roche's call to action. I understood the medical part. I knew of the need. But what didn't make sense was the business part. We knew from all our presentations that American pharmaceutical companies did not see the value of an automated diagnostic. Being North American and EU–centric, they saw no real prospect for profit elsewhere. To them, the rest of the world was a giveaway, a charity, not an economic gain but a net cost. It might be a goodwill gesture, but not a successful business venture. After all, medicine in the developing world would yield pennies on the dollar. Besides, who wants a family of tests like HER2 that single out (target) a subset of patients? Better to treat the denominator than the numerator. These companies saw us as diminishing the prospects of blockbuster drugs. In retrospect, we had been casting pearls to swine.

This begged the question, What did the Swiss see that the Americans didn't? Why buy a diagnostic company to globalize the testing in the rest of the world if you would only lose money? Were the Swiss missionaries, or possibly savvy in a way unseen by the Americans? Or perhaps both? And so I reiterated to Franz and Severin, "The US companies see the rest of the world outside the EU as a loss. Why do you see it differently?"

My perplexity was short lived. Globalization as they saw it was not the liability; it was the key. Severin explained.

"You have been given a very North American–centric answer. Yes, they are right, North America and the EU are the economic Mount Everest of drug sales, but they have their limitations."

"Really?" I was intrigued. "How?"

"Well, North America is 4 percent of the world's population and the EU is 5 percent, which leaves 91 percent of the global population as our potential market."

"But what about the economic factor? Our prices are high and profitable in North America and the EU, but they will not hold up elsewhere."

Then came Severin's surprise answer. "The price is the same everywhere." And, as I smirked, he finished the sentence. "But we can help."

He went on to explain that the value of the test was the same all over the world, and we should actively sell that value, thereby protecting the worldwide price. But where necessary, we might pay the second half of it—thereby being charitable as an end, not a beginning. I can say after going to more than a hundred countries, Severin's strategy proved correct. With his prompting, we learned to sell value over price, and it worked, even in developing countries.

Another factor that boosted our value selling was the Roche global infrastructure. Their century-long global presence with service engineers and support staff in every country was a major plus. Remember our Libyan doctor who called me to the booth to praise her Roche support staff. That was an important part of her value equation.

And so began our pursuit of the 91 percent; so began our globalization, our journeying to Tunisia, Turkey, Thailand, and anywhere and everywhere HER2-positive invasive breast cancer patients might be found. Suddenly, geography mattered. After all, is a thirty-eight-year-old woman with HER2-positive breast cancer in need of the Roche Herceptin* any different in Botswana than Boston, in Buenos Aires than Boise? Our mission became find her, diagnose her, and treat her.

Besides driving globalization and economic growth, there was one other major positive result from the acquisition. When Roche bought Ventana, it was the first time a pharmaceutical company bought a pathology company. By investing in this marriage of the diagnostic to the therapeutic, Roche immediately revalued pathology *and* the pathologist. They asked the diagnostician to go beyond mere classification to explaining the nature of the disease, to identifying the target of therapy. They asked pathologists to raise the bar and to produce more actionable personal results. They encouraged pathologists to practice personalized medicine.

At this writing, ten years on, Ventana has grown in revenue per annum from $290 million in 2007 to $1.2 billion in 2018, up

330 percent. And the anti-HER2 drug Herceptin* went from $3 billion in revenues in 2007 to north of $7 billion in 2017. Also, we have gone from twenty countries to more than a hundred and have added six more FDA-approved tests relevant to targeted therapy. By any measure, whether economic or medical, the Swiss and Roche calculated correctly and wisely.

We generally experienced win-win capitalism. That is, there was a win at every level, from inventor, to employee, to medical doctor, to patient, to investor. First, the inventors were given the time and capital to invent. Second, the employees were given the means to build, sell, support, and refine that product. Third, the medical doctors were given new tools and capabilities to improve diagnosis and treatment. Fourth, the patients were given more certain diagnoses and more informed treatments. Fifth, the new capabilities—valuable to doctors *and* their patients—gave increased economic value to the investors, both venture capitalists and shareholders, which was realized by growing revenue, increasing stock prices, and ultimately by a high monetary return upon acquisition.

It was win-win and defined the true virtue of proper, principled long-term capitalism. Money was used to invent and build new products, to transform medicine, and to create economic return, and gains would be harvested for further transformative projects.

Although we generally enjoyed this virtuous form of capitalism, we also sometimes saw the non-virtuous side. We sometimes saw the compulsion to profit disproportionately, and inappropriately. We saw the desire for excessive gain, for inequitable, inordinate gain.

Yes, occasionally greed did find us. One instance comes to mind, and to quote Lin-Manuel Miranda, I was "in the room when it happened."

The room where it happened was a conference room in our law firm's offices in downtown Chicago. It was early January in 2008. The Ventana Board of Directors, myself included, were meeting to finalize the details of the impending acquisition by Roche. We were sequestered with our Ventana business-development team, our Chicago legal team, and one of our investment banking teams. We'd just been through a seven-month rollercoaster ride of a hostile takeover. The goal was to agree to some details of the transaction, seek a resolution, and agree to the acquisition. Some of it was dotting the *i*'s and crossing the *t*'s, but it also involved substantial matters like setting the purchase price, detailing the assets to be transferred, e.g., the plant in Tucson and the intellectual property, and accounting for our obligations, such as debts and payments due to others.

Although there were differences of opinion, the overall mood was of relief and satisfaction; we were discharging our fiduciary duty to the shareholders. We were soon to give them hard-earned, appropriate financial gain in uncertain financial times, this being early 2008, just before the Great Recession.

Some of our to-be-paid obligations were at the table, including our legal team and our investment bankers. In both cases, we had a contract to cover their time and effort. As our chairman, Jack Schuler, reminded us of these obligations, the board members all nodded in affirmation, understanding payment was soon due. While the legal team nodded along with us, one of our banking teams was quick to suggest that, given the likely very favorable outcome—a soon-to-be executed $3.4-billion deal—a bonus might be in order.

They suggested that a previously agreed-upon $10-million contract amount might be appropriately upped to $25 million or $30 million, given the purchase price was likely to top $3 billion. They thought that a bonus closer to 1 percent of the amount of the deal was appropriate.

This had not been an agenda item, so Jack Schuler, our chairman, asked that they step out into the hallway while we discussed the matter.

As soon as they left, after minimal discussion, the board of directors voted a unanimous negative. The general sentiment was that a deal was a deal. The contracted $10 million seemed reasonable for the seven-month effort. They did an excellent job serving as the negotiator and the marriage broker, but a deal was a deal.

When I looked around the room, the unanimous negative vote was predictable. If the nine board of directors members had one thing in common, it was that we were all self-made men. All had toiled for every penny. Yes, some had received bonuses, but as agreed upon before, not after the fact.

In addition to myself, there was Ed Giles, the old school, principled, white-shoe, Ivy League Wall Street investor. There was Jim Bates, the distinguished long-term investor of Allstate Insurance funds, who had been making astute investments generating consistent growth for forty years. There were, of course, John Patience and Jack Schuler, who had not only invested heavily in Ventana, but given it countless hours of nearly daily attention. There was Jim Weersing, the Stanford engineer, who had worked with Hewlett and Packard and was then leading a venture fund following the ever-honest "HP way." There was Rod Dammeyer, the always-savvy tech company investor, who knew medical device companies like a well-schooled savant. And, finally, there were Tom Brown and Mark Miller, who had worked for Jack at Abbott and knew of his straight-dealing ways.

Also, Mark was the CEO in another Schuler/Patience company, Stericycle, bringing it from nothing to number one in hospital waste management.

These were all men who realized economic gain by their own hands-on toil, not simply by financial cunning. They were accustomed to investing in new inventions and products to transform the workplace, not simply to boost their own net worth.

Jack was soon next door to diplomatically communicate our appreciation for their job well done, but a deal was a deal. Thank you very much.

A few minutes later, Jack returned to say that our banker heard us loud and clear but wanted us to understand a fact we might not appreciate. Namely, that the requested bonus could be paid in Swiss francs, not US dollars, since the simple fact was Roche was now acquiring not only our assets but also our obligations. So if we now, as the still-governing board of directors, included this obligation on the list, the Swiss would ultimately be obliged to pay, not us. They urged us to consider that fact.

Once again, the discussion was short and the vote unanimous in the negative. We each saw it the same way; whether Ventana or Roche, dollars or Swiss francs, it was still shareholder money and not to be given away without regard to our fiduciary responsibility.

It was too sly, too slick, too much sleight of hand for us. It felt reptilian, as in slithering and furtive.

Jack was soon back in the other room, again diplomatically rejecting their logic.

When he returned a few minutes later he advised us of another of the banker's perspectives. They wanted us to understand that for the multiple Ventana investors, and the venture capitalists in particular, our penuriousness might make it difficult for us to work with them in future transactions. Did we understand?

This time the vote was even faster, and less diplomatic.

"No, no, no . . . Consequences be damned!"

And so it happened that nothing sly, nothing cunning, and nothing damaging to the shareholders, be they American or Swiss, occurred that day. All it took was a simple "no." Greed averted.

There was nothing in writing, nothing but a fleeting moment. Nothing bad came of it. But as I was in the room where it happened, I came to understand how excessive reward and cunning, sly, furtive financial transactions can occur as simply as a serpent slithers into the brush.

Recollecting this account of what she called *bad capitalism*, Mom reminded me that not all the characters in my thirty-year tale were worthy of the assembly of like souls. Some fell short.

With the acquisition complete, the integration began. It was partly a marriage of culture and of business practice. The social integration had an excitement to it, just as finding new friends makes life interesting. There was an ease to it as both companies had a common purpose, and even though it was a business transaction, it wasn't all serious business.

As we began to travel between Tucson and Basel, we came to learn some of the joys of being Swiss. We learned of the pleasure of a wood-fired cheesy Emmental-laced *raclette*, of a crisp potato rösti, of a walnut honey *engadiner nusstorte*, and the joy of Sprüngli chocolates.

As more and more Swiss came from Basel to Tucson, we familiarized them with the joys of hominy-rich pozole stew, carne asada–filled chimichangas, and poblano-laced quesadillas, and cinnamon-sugary churros.

Between Switzerland and Arizona, we had the mountains and trekking in common, although we did have to teach the Swiss how to deal with our desert critters. So, orientation included tips on how to avoid javelinas, rattlesnakes, scorpions, and Gila monsters. We also alerted them to botanical hazards not found trekking in the Alps, like jumping cholla, prickly pear cactus, thorny ocotillo and—worst of all—the spiked agave known as shin daggers.

In general, the social integration went swimmingly well. The biggest change was to be the magnitude and reach of our business. In order to become a global company, in order to go everywhere on the planet, we needed to learn from the Swiss, who had been out there with pharmaceuticals and medical devices for more than a hundred years. It was time to adjust and learn new ways. As we went from twenty countries to one hundred, from manufacturing hundreds to thousands of instruments, from producing small lots to gigantic lots of reagents, we needed to achieve Swiss precision. We needed to be more thorough in our planning, and more predictable and reliable in our manufacturing.

We came at our new obligations with all the daring and exuberance of a startup, but it was time to be less free-wheeling and more disciplined. We needed to tick with the precision of a fine Swiss watch. To this end, we focused heavily on the need to build more reliable, durable, transportable products.

Besides these internal improvements, the acquisition brought us new capabilities. With the added capital and business heft of Roche, we were able to greatly expand our capabilities by external acquisition.

We had started down that path before the Swiss, having acquired an antibody-producing company, Spring, to ensure we had world-class antibodies. The Swiss then gave us a much greater capacity to expand our scientific capabilities. With Roche support, we acquired a digital image-analysis company, Bioimagene, which would allow computer analysis, quantification, and transmission of our visual microscopic results to others. This was to lead to a new Roche report-generating system known as Navify.

But beyond getting up to speed on the Swiss approach to process precision and doing business on a global scale, we learned the sacrosanct importance of punctuality, the societal reverence for hierarchy, and the rules that underpin civility. We also had to learn a new corporate language replete with an alphabet soup of acronyms. For example, the agenda for a meeting would have sessions featuring the CEC, PBM, and DBM, covering topics ranging from PHC to NMEs, BLAs, LIPs, and IVDs (translation for the uninitiated: corporate executive committee, pharma business meeting, diagnostics business meeting, personalized healthcare, new molecular entities, biologics license applications, lifecycle investment points, and in-vitro diagnostics). To be fair, all large corporations are no doubt afflicted with their own strains of the acronym virus, but Roche's seemed particularly virulent.

In spite of any and all challenges—from the nine-hour time-zone difference that sometimes required us Tucson colleagues to participate in conference calls at odd hours, to getting used to a new set of acronyms and corporate terms, to the sometimes time-consuming and frustrating Swiss reliance on consensus—being acquired by Roche was one of the best things that ever happened to Ventana, and it opened the door to experiences, relationships, and perspectives that dramatically enriched my life and those of many of my colleagues. And that holds true to this day.

A second acquisition brought us to a broader global challenge. Roche, through the acquisition of MTM Laboratories in Heidelberg, Germany, brought us to the global problem of cervical cancer. This cancer is a serious widespread problem resulting in 311,000 deaths per year with 90 percent of those deaths occurring in poor countries. To solve the problem required global reach and hundreds of millions of dollars. The imperative to act came from the fact that this was a preventable disease and therefore global eradication was possible.

To eradicate the disease would require new tools.

This need was met by MTM's development of a new immunocytochemical (ICC) test—the dual P16/Ki-67 test—which readily detected precancerous cells. P16 is a cellular protein that functions to impede cell division, and Ki-67 is a marker for rapid cell division. Think of the P16 as the brakes and Ki-67 as the accelerator. Usually a normal cell is either stopping or going. How could it do both at once? That is abnormal and pathologic. Another way to think of it is to imagine coming to an intersection and finding both the red and green lights are on. Clearly, the traffic light is broken. And so it is with the precancerous cells; if both P16 (red) and Ki-67 (green) are present in the same cell, that cell is broken. It is diseased. It is pathologically deranged. Do not proceed. Stop and remove.

This dual test was a first in diagnostic medicine. It showed there is a chemistry to precancerous change at the level of cell function and that using ICC we could visualize that altered chemistry, that altered function.

As it turned out, not only was this dual positive ICC test better at predicting precancer and cancer than the standard PAP test, but also—very importantly—a dual negative ICC test result gave a better reassurance that a cancer would not develop over the next few years. This meant that an ICC-negative woman could wait three years before being screened again, in contrast with the historic norm of required one-year follow-up.

The consequence of the improved testing accuracy was fewer unnecessary procedures, fewer hospitalizations, and fewer follow-up clinic visits. It resulted in a measurable improvement in both patient well-being and in medical costs. It speaks to the power of disease prevention and the utility of protein (ICC) testing to improve testing accuracy.

Understanding that we could play a role in cancer prevention had a profound effect on our understanding of our mission. For these patients, our goal shifted from *improving* the lives of all patients afflicted with cancer to *preventing* the affliction. It was understanding we could allow the diagnostician to be the up-front guy, not the after-the-fact guy. Remember Bill Doyle?

This medical practice–changing dual ICC test was developed in Heidelberg by Ruediger Ridder and his team at MTM through a multiyear effort. The MTM company was acquired by Roche in 2011. After a twelve-year effort with clinical trials, MTM's p16 biomarker had achieved a World Health Organization (WHO) recommendation of favoring the p16 test over the then-standard test. You could say Ruediger had invented a new field of diagnostics—the field of dysfunctional cellular pathology. He uniquely perceived that to see at the level of cellular function would allow new insight into the beginning of disease, and the power of seeing the beginning was being able to prevent subsequent progression. Ruediger's dual stain viewed in a microscope made precancer visible and actionable in a way that anyone, even Gaddafi, could see.

Ruediger was driven to understand what Sir Francis Bacon called "the secret motion of things and the knowledge of causes." This is the same mindset that Binford had back in Cebu that turned me to pathology.

After the MTM acquisition, Ruediger and I had adjacent offices and as fellow founders of a startup had a common bond and became kindred spirits. We were like rare birds of the same feather, say two bristlehead shrikes, meeting in the vastness of the Borneo jungle.

Most founders vanish after acquisition; after all, who wants to go from the top position to being just one of 95,000 employees? But we both stayed. We saw it similarly. Having birthed the child, we wanted to stick with it to ensure our baby would make it out of the nursery, come of age, and travel the world. To do otherwise seemed an abandonment.

Ruediger understood that his dual test, even with its WHO recommendation as the new standard of care, needed the Ventana automation to make it everywhere. Accordingly, we both stuck to parenting and coaching over the ensuing decade.

As time passed, we both took the unconventional view that we could foster a startup mentality within the larger company. For him, MTM kept that pioneering spirit going, and for me, it was a group within Ventana I called Medical Innovation, which kept our blue-sky mentality alive. After all, big companies need blue sky, too!

Mom, having had an annual PAP smear each of the last seventy years, had an abiding interest in the matter of the dual ICC test, which might mean fewer clinic visits, fewer procedures, and better care. As she said, "How about twenty to twenty-five visits rather than seventy?"

She marveled at Ruediger, who had persisted for eighteen years, from the initial development of the dual test, through the clinical trials, to the necessary FDA approvals. As she said, "He is amazing. He persisted for eighteen years to become an overnight success!"

She had questions for me about the why and the how of it all. Why did the clinical trials take so long? How much did Roche spend? And if the treatment was surgical and there was no drug involved, how would Roche ever get a return on their investment?

I explained the timing. Because they had to prove a negative—a cancer that was prevented and did not recur—and because it takes years for that cancer to either recur or not, the clinical studies took five to ten years and required tens of thousands of patients at hundreds of medical testing and treating sites. As for the money, the expense ran into the hundreds of millions, perhaps to half a billion, as the trials involved so many patients at so many sites over so much time. And there was the price of acquiring MTM. As for the return on investment, given that Roche had no follow-on therapeutic, well, that might take twenty to twenty-five years.

Mom's last question. "Why would a business invest so much and choose to lose money for so long?"

"Well, I believe they saw it as a global problem that could be solved. They saw 311,000 deaths that were preventable. They saw a disease that could be eradicated, and they had the intellectual and scientific means and the motivation to do so. They understood that to change medicine globally requires a willingness to invest heavily beyond immediate gain. I think they felt a social responsibility."

As a retired librarian at a public library with a keen social conscience, Mom liked that answer and was pleased to welcome Ruediger and Roche into her assembly of like souls.

One major consequence of the acquisition was the ratcheting up of our global travel. On the path to one hundred countries, we were all in the air all the time. By the fourth year, we'd reached twenty-seven countries. This, added to my twenty-two prior years of travel, brought me to the seven-million-mile mark—with all twenty-two spent in steerage at the back of the plane.

Our collective mission was to make a global market. We were out to change medicine in every city, in every country in the world. That was the high-minded positive side. The negative side was the psychological and physical challenge of constant, time zone–crossing travel.

International travel quickly loses its glamor when every stop on a ten-stop trip of 18,000 miles is spent in a stuffy conference room, listening to the sound of your own voice. After eight to ten days of this, the only thought is of home. That yearning for home all too often turned to agony as return flights were thwarted by mechanical or weather delays. I remember one instance in particular, a trip to Berlin that took place in the dead of an ice-cold winter in 2012.

The travelers were me, who we will call the veteran with seven million miles, and rookie David Chaffin, a Ventana scientist on his first overseas trip. The occasion was a prestigious scientific meeting at the Charité Hospital at Humboldt University in the former East Berlin. We were excited to be there for two reasons. First, Charité was the birthplace of pathology. We would present in the very same anatomical theatre where Professor Rudolph Virchow founded our field 160 years before. Second, all the top European professors were there, and it was our chance to impress the thought leaders. It was our opportunity to make an intellectual market.

As it turned out, the trip to Berlin had expected and unexpected outcomes. As intended, the rookie scientist, David, presented his data at the academic forum held at the Charité. The rookie presented three years of data in thirty minutes and did a brilliant job. His findings were well received by the top professors. The enthusiasm of the thought leaders was a well-deserved boost and a reward for his prior effort. This recognition came on the heels of the three patent filings we had made back home—that's how significant his work was.

So for the rookie, it was mission accomplished. Well done, as intended.

Now for the unexpected bit. The day after the academic meeting, we were at Berlin's Tegel Airport, ready to return to Arizona, when a snowy whiteout canceled all flights. The next available flight out was three days later. The rookie, hoping to get home for his son's birthday, was apoplectic. The veteran immediately jumped into action. Using my iPhone weather app, I determined that the Hamburg airport one hundred and seventy five miles away was yet snow free, so I hatched a plan to take a train to Hamburg and get the Ventana/Roche travel agent back in Indianapolis to find a flight out the next day. While HQ was working on next-day flights, the veteran and the rookie hopped a taxi to catch a train.

In the taxi, the rookie was showing signs of stress in the category of a cold sweat. The veteran, reading the rookie's anxiety, inquired about his labored breathing

"Are you alright?" the veteran asked.

"Not really."

"Why?"

"I am very uneasy about our plan," the rookie admitted.

"What makes you uneasy?"

"We're in a taxi to a train station of uncertain location, to take a train that we don't know will be there, to a city where we do not yet have a room, in order to get up tomorrow and catch a flight on which we have no seat. That's all." The rookie accentuated his words with repeated twitches and wiggles.

"Is that all?" the veteran replied.

The pair arrived at the station at 3:01 p.m. to see there was indeed a 3:15 to Hamburg. The veteran was elated; the rookie was still twitching.

"What good luck we have a train!" the veteran said.

"What bad luck we don't have tickets," the rookie retorted.

"What good luck I see the ticket office nearby."

"What bad luck there is a long line for tickets and just one clerk."

"What good luck there's an automated ticket booth."

The rookie was unimpressed. "What bad luck it's only in German, no English."

Again, the veteran jumped into action, feeding a credit card into the automated ticket machine and quickly mashing the buttons, completely unwitting of the German instructions. The veteran played the machine like a Vegas slot machine, but alas, no three cherries and no tickets. The time was 3:09 when the rookie sought the help of a nearby stranger who kindly pushed two buttons, yielding two tickets to Hamburg on the 3:15. After a dash to the platform, our two travelers were safely aboard, off to Hamburg, thanks to the kindness of a stranger and the rookie chipping in to save the veteran.

Fast-forward two hours, they arrived in Hamburg, and headquarters came through. Situation as follows: destination reached, hotel room found, plane tickets secured. Within the hour, check-in was complete and all arrangements were made. The veteran and the rookie were off to a *Hofbräu*, and after tucking away a few pints and a few brats, the rookie began to warm to the pleasures of business travel and the joy of obstacles overcome. The veteran was now feeling smug; after all, the next set of obstacles was a day away.

All in all, it's a good thing the rookie had the veteran to get him through the obstacles. And for the veteran, it was good he had the rookie to deliver the science and carry his bags.

Mom found the 3:15 to Hamburg amusing and had a good chuckle. I knew it was quite civilized compared to her travels in Africa. It was mild compared to her narrow-gauge rail journey into upland Liberia, which ended in a jungle trek by foot to a remote village to visit Peace Corps friends. It was mild compared to her and Dad's bumpy ride on a motorbike on the rutted streets of Kizimkazi in Zanzibar, with overly zealous Chicoms hot on their tails.

16.

Slaying Serpents

OVER FORTY YEARS, THE DIAGNOSIS and treatment of cancer has realized two spectacular insights. First, cancer often is not characterized by a single abnormality; it may evolve into a multi-headed beast, requiring multiple adaptive treatments. Second, the multi-headed beast has another therapy-confounding trick of becoming invisible to the body's immune response by putting up a force field requiring new drugs—immunotherapy—to overcome the blockade.

As we have learned, to eliminate a cancer, you must eliminate the last immortalized cell. To kill that cell, you must know the nature of the beast. You must know its workings, its derangements, its dependencies, its driving force. The driving force may then become the target of a drug, making a knockout punch possible. And repeated treatment with the targeted drug over time will deal with any dormancy issue.

These principles underlie personalized targeted therapy. But what if the beast has more than one driving force? What if the beast is a multi-headed serpent, like the Hydra? What if when you lop off one head, as Hercules did in Greek mythology, another springs forth? What if the serpent evolves and grows more heads as you

treat? What if the drug itself stimulates new heads? What if the
serpent has the capacity to change like a chameleon? What then?
Our next patient is a case in point.

In the spring of 2005, our forty-year-old patient Tom Weiser
was found to have fifteen lung tumors. These were likely metastases
of his colon cancer, which had been removed a year before. After
surgery, Tom was treated with chemotherapy. His colon cancer was
positive for an epidermal growth factor receptor—EGFR HER1,
which is similar to HER2—and so he also received an anti-EGFR
drug (Erlotinib). But within months he relapsed with lung metastasis.

The situation was dire. The advice was to treat with fragmented
ion-beam radiation. While the radiation worked on most of the
tumors, five remained unphased. For these, the recommendation
was for add-on, salvage chemotherapy, a form of palliative treatment.
Palliation was the only choice since a cure, he was told, was out of
the question. His question then was, "How long do I have?" The
answer from his oncologist was six to nine months, max.

Unwilling to surrender, he asked, "Why just palliate? Why not
go for the cure by surgical removal?" He sought a thoracic surgeon's
opinion. The answer—tumor plucking is out of the question for
three reasons. First, given their location, tucked in near major blood
vessels, it would require a thoracotomy. That would involve cracking
open his chest by splitting his breastbone and opening him up like a
Thanksgiving turkey. Second, there was no guarantee that all five spots
could be plucked, given they were small and scattered. Third, tumor
plucking had long been abandoned as futile with no history of success.

Facing a hopeless situation, Tom followed a different logic and
came to a different conclusion. He reasoned that if his initial colon
cancer was EGFR-driven and the anti-EGFR drug had knocked
it back, then the recurrence must mean the tumor was driven by

something other than EGFR. So, he wanted his chest cracked and the tumors removed. Even if you can't get all five, we could at least see what this chameleon has become, he concluded. This was risky business, and certainly not standard practice at the time.

Tom, by this logic, defying medical convention and against medical advice, pushed for and received his wish for a thoracotomy. As it turned out, the surgeon was right; only three spots could be removed, so cure by this means was not possible. But by another measure, Tom was also right. The three plucked tumors were "something other." They were not EGFR over-expressive. They were heavily expressive of IGFR, a different growth factor. The tumor had indeed evolved to another driving force. It had evolved to thrive by other means. It had survived as a chameleon does, by changing its color.

As fate would have it, at that time there was a new anti-IGFR drug in a phase II clinical trial, and Tom was to become one of only two patients out of twenty-five to respond to this new drug, with all his tumor spots resolving. And so, between the anti-IGFR drug and the radiotherapy, the cascade of metastatic tumors was stopped, and time was bought.

Astoundingly, over time, Tom was to have seven more recurrences. Each time, they were pulmonary, each time they changed color, each time a targeted drug had at least a partial effect. Enough to prolong his life for more than nine years, far beyond the six to nine months he was first given.

While the combination of polypharmacy, surgery, and radiotherapy prolonged his life, it also multiplied his side effects. He was eventually worn to a debilitating state, suffering from constant nausea, diarrhea, gnawing pain, hair loss, and a beet-red, oozing rash.

It was at this low point, when he was seemingly at the end of his therapeutic tether, I asked Tom how he could bear to go on. His answer, "Whatever it takes to go for a cure, even if just to buy time to the next breakthrough. If not, I have a wife and four kids [ages seven to fourteen], and I want to see them grow, succeed, and graduate from college." His goal was to be cured, but his fallback was to endure, hope for a breakthrough, and see his family grow and succeed. And so, highly motivated as he was, he persevered well beyond any conventional expectations.

Then in the eighth year, there came what seemed a big breakthrough. In his seventh recurrence, we found a mutation (BRAF V600E) for which there was a new anti-BRAF drug (Vemurafenib). He was then treated with the combination of that drug and an anti-EGFR drug (Erlotinib). The effect was miraculous. There was a seemingly complete remission. There was jubilation. Champagne was sipped as Tom and his family celebrated a breakthrough at last.

Yet, shockingly, twelve weeks later, Tom died of metastasis to his brain. The combination had worked on his lung, but not his brain, on the other side of the impermeable blood-brain barrier. Tom's brain metastasis predicted death within the month, but Tom, out of sheer willpower, was to fight on. In the end, he died two days after his eldest daughter, Emily, graduated from the University of Arizona. He died knowing she succeeded, knowing his family was well. He died knowing he had given all he had.

Beyond himself and his family, Tom taught his physicians lessons not found in textbooks. He taught them that tumors may be heterogeneous, that tumors evolve, and that the phenotypic (protein status) and genotypic (gene status) details of every biopsy are needed to identify targets of therapy. He taught them not to give up on patients who fail therapy. He taught them how much we can learn from individual patients who are the first ones into phase I and II trials. We practice conventional standard-of-care medicine based on population studies, but we learn of game-changing possibilities from remarkable patients like Tom who have the courage and daring to endure great difficulty and produce improbable results.

Years later, trying to make sense of Tom Weiser's travail, seeking to understand the nature of his beast, I made a schematic summary of his many recurrences, focusing on his myriad phenotypic and genotypic findings (see Fig. 6). They appear as an ever-branching tree. I summarized the corresponding targeted drugs that were used to trim the branches. In retrospect, although trimming the branches was well informed by our repeated study of his recurrences, and while it certainly prolonged his life, cure was not possible because we were dealing with the mythological Hydra, and as Hercules learned 2,500 years ago, lopping off one head at a time will not kill it (see fig. 7). Perhaps it would be better in the future to forego the heads and go for the collective, underlying body. As we will learn with our next and last patient, that stratagem was to come to bear in the form of immunotherapy, some two years after Tom died. Tom was right again in his motivation to live long enough for the next breakthrough.

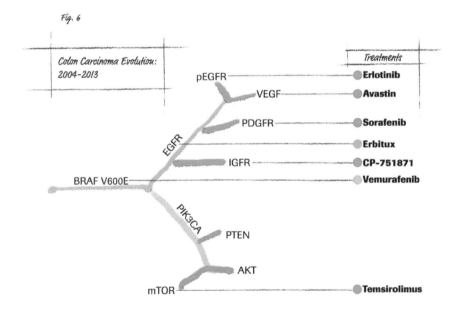

Fig. 6. Tom Weiser's colon carcinoma evolution from 2004 to 2013. This is a schematic summary of Tom's many recurrences. With each recurrence, we found a new gene status (genotype) and a new protein status (phenotype) for his mutations. This evolution of Tom's tumors appears as an ever-branching tree. To the right, I summarized the corresponding targeted drugs that were used to "trim the branches."

Fig. 7

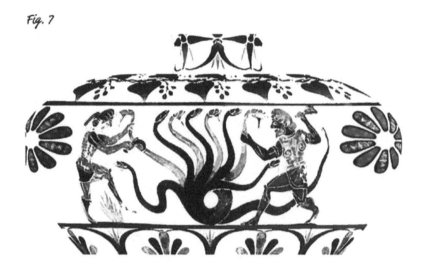

Fig. 7. Detail of painted terra-cotta water jar (Etruscan, 520–510 BC) showing Hercules preparing to lop off a head as he battles the multiheaded serpent, the Hydra. (Digital image courtesy of the Getty's Open Content Program.)

To access image:

http://www.getty.edu/art/collection/objects/10600/attributed-to-eagle-painter-caeretan-hydria-etruscan-caeretan-520-510-bc/?dz=#41436c7a1165de e16e7d39bb484c77bc1460a949

Hearing me through, Mom reminded me that I had told only half of Tom's story. I had told of his medical journey, but not of his more vibrant personal story. As she pointed out, Tom taught more than his physicians; he taught all Ventana how to fight. And so the untold story began.

Tom Weiser was a long-time Ventana employee serving as our North American field customer relations manager. He was a naturally funny, exuberant, and engaging person. He was a fighter, and he never stopped fighting his disease, nor did he ever stop making people smile. He was a profound influence on the whole company.

Among countless inspirational moments with Tom over the years, three stand out.

First, at the end of his life in the weeks before he died, just after surgery to remove his brain metastasis, I asked him how he could bear the constant pain. He answered me with a baseball story about the 1986 College World Series (CWS). Tom was there in Omaha, Nebraska, as the student manager of the University of Arizona baseball team. As he recalled, "We were playing Maine. We were down 7–0 in the seventh inning and facing certain elimination. But with a lot of hustle and a few mighty swings of the bat we won 8–7 and then ended up winning the CWS and being named national champions." Then he continued. "I see this the same way. It is only going to take one swing of the bat to knock this thing out of my body. I just need to keep swinging until I can't swing anymore."

Second, there was the time with Tom at our annual sales meeting in Dallas. On that occasion, Beck Weathers, a pathologist from Dallas, was the keynote speaker. He described for us his near-death experience on Mount Everest in 1996. As detailed by Jon Krakauer in his book, *Into Thin Air*, Beck was left for dead three times, thought to be one of seven others who had died that day. Left hypothermic in a subzero blizzard overnight, he somehow rose the next morning and stumbled back to camp, severely frostbitten but alive. He described that moment lying helpless in the snow, that last flicker of life. As he put it, "I was struggling to keep the pilot light on, and the thought of my wife and family were the faint flame that wouldn't go out."

After his talk, I interviewed Tom about his ongoing cancer fight. As we chatted informally on the stage in two easy chairs before an audience of 300 Ventana marketing and sales employees, I said to Tom, "It strikes me that your experience is similar to Beck's. You have both climbed a daunting mountain and you have both been near death." Tom replied, "Yes and no. Yes, we have both climbed a daunting mountain and have faced death, and both of us drew strength from our families. But there are two key differences. First, Beck chose that mountain. I didn't choose mine; it chose me. Second, he nearly died three times—I have nearly died seven times." He said this matter-of-factly, without an iota of bitterness.

In his nine-year battle, Tom continued to work at his Ventana job through his treatments, his surgeries, and his recurrences. He worked up to the end. He credited his wife, Heidi, their four children, and his faith for his strength. He held on beyond the overwhelming odds against him and only surrendered a few days after his daughter Emily graduated from the University of Arizona.

In those nine years, we kept Tom on the full payroll and did not place him on disability till the very end. He was too important. He was too valuable. We needed him in the dugout when we were down 7–0. As Tom fought, so did we. He was to become a pillar of our cultural beliefs. He was the guy all knew and admired, who taught us how to endure with unabated enthusiasm.

The third and last occasion was Tom's funeral in Sacramento near his home in Roseville, California. On this solemn occasion, Ventana employees from all over the country flew in to pay their respects. There was no obligation to attend; there was only a deep sense that we as a company had become a true family, and that Tom was the very soul of that family. It was Tom who taught us that a company can have a soul, and a company with a soul is capable of greatness, as Tom Weiser was.

On September 29, 2015, a seventy-year-old sat in the waiting room of the oncology clinic at UCLA in Los Angeles. He held two objects. In one hand, a clear plastic case with five microscopic slides, and in the other an iPad. He was waiting to see Dr. Antoni Ribas, the world-renowned expert on treating malignant melanoma.

Our seventy-year-old was there for a second opinion. In question was not his diagnosis. The microscopic slides he brought showed a nasty malignant melanoma had invaded deeply into his scalp and metastasized to the adjacent lymph nodes. These facts were established unequivocally six weeks before. Also not in question was the nature of the disease, as the iPad he brought showed all the scans and all the chemistry performed over the previous six weeks.

The chemistry showed both the phenotype (protein status) and genotype (gene status) of the melanoma. The genotype, done by next-generation sequencing (NGS), detailed fourteen separate mutations, indicating a hyper-mutated tumor. That was definitively a multi-headed beast, another Hydra. As Hercules learned the hard way, lopping off one head would not kill it.

Finally, not in question was another critical factor—the extent of the disease. This was well established after three surgeries and four scans. The three surgeries were: first, the local excision of the tumor, a pea-sized bump on the top of the patient's head with several surrounding bumps (satellitosis); second, the removal of a nearby sentinel node for biopsy; and the third was a neck dissection seeking further lymph-node involvement. The first surgery showed a deep-seated melanoma, a malignancy of pigment-bearing skin cells, the second a positive lymph node, and the third revealed forty-five nodes all negative for melanoma.

After the surgeries, multiple scans revealed no evidence of melanoma. According to all the facts considered and documented on the iPad, his was unequivocally a stage IIIB malignant melanoma with no further evidence of disease (NED) post-surgery.

The question for Dr. Ribas was what should be done to improve the odds, given that stage IIIB melanoma with satellitosis has an 80 percent recurrence rate, that recurrences are uniformly fatal, and that his previous oncologists' opinions were that he should just go home and wait and see?

It turned out, what our seventy-year-old and Dr. Ribas had in common that day was that neither were wait-and-see guys. Our seventy-year old was more of a give-it-everything-you've-got guy. And Dr. Ribas, who had seen a lot of melanoma patients die over the years, was more of an out-to-change-the-odds guy. What brought our seventy-year-old to the waiting room that day was that Dr. Ribas had just published an amazing medical paper in *Nature*, a top scientific journal, describing an extraordinary result treating end-stage melanoma with a new approach (immunotherapy) that harnessed the body's own immune system to fight cancer using a new drug called Keytruda˚ made by Merck (Tumeh, P. C., et al. pp. 568–571).

This new approach was based on boosting the patient's own immune-cell response to eliminate their cancer. The idea was to strengthen the body's lymphocytes (CD8-positive T cells), the wolves of the immune system, to induce self-healing. The surprise was the discovery—for which James Allison and Tasuku Honjo won a Nobel Prize in October 2018—that cancer cells often confound the self-healing response by putting up a molecular blockade (PD-L1), a cloak of invisibility that keeps the wolves at bay. Knowing this, big pharma companies synthesized a whole new generation of drugs (anti-PD-L1) like Keytruda˚ to block the blockage, remove the invisible cloak, and allow self-healing.

Our seventy-year-old brought a plastic container that held the glass microscope slide that showed his melanoma was strongly PD-L1-positive. As he and Dr. Ribas sat together at the microscope, the PD-L1 blockade was obvious. They also saw the tumor was surrounded—but not yet invaded—by CD8-positive T cells (see Fig. 8). The blockade was indeed keeping the wolves at bay. This was the very constellation of change that Dr. Ribas had seen before in his patients who responded to the immunotherapy agent Keytruda˚.

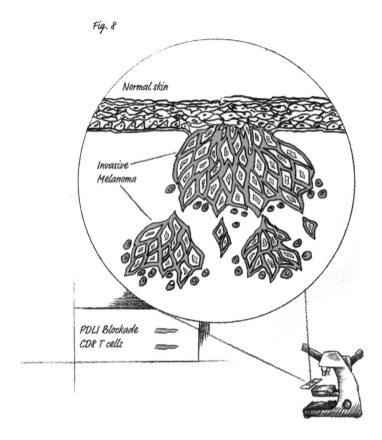

Fig. 8. The "last patient's" biopsy, showing an invasive malignant melanoma with immune blockade (blue) preventing self-healing by the CD8-immune T cells (red).

Just as the two became animated, Dr. Ribas stopped suddenly and turned to address a third party—the seventy-year-old's wife of fifty years—also in the room.

"Sorry," he said. "Your husband being an academic MD, we quickly jumped into the detail without explaining to you." Then, bringing her to the scope, he explained.

"We are seeing both the tumor and the immune response. We are seeing the lay of the land, the battlefield between tumor and host, and we now need to change the landscape. The blockade is keeping the wolves at bay, and it's time to unleash them. It's time to invoke some immune self-healing."

While explaining the favorable prospect for targeted immunotherapy using Keytruda˚, Dr. Ribas was quick to point out two very significant obstacles. The first, surgery had removed all evidence of melanoma, which the scans confirmed, so as he said, "If we treat, there will be no visible tumor to observe and measure."

Before he could go on, the wife interrupted. "I know, I know. You're chasing the invisible. Been there, done that."

Surprised, Dr. Ribas asked, "How is that?"

"Well," she continued, "ten years ago I had a diffuse large B-cell lymphoma, and my oncologist said to cure me he had to get to the last cell—and to do that, we had to chase the invisible. That was the famous Dr. Tom Miller at the University of Arizona. Do you know him?"

"Before my time, but you're right, we will be chasing the invisible."

She interrupted again, serving as her husband's protector. "What is the second obstacle?"

"Well, unlike with lymphoma, targeted therapy—immunotherapy—is not yet given up front as adjunctive therapy for melanoma. There is no national study available. I am writing one now, but implementation will take years."

The seventy-year-old anxiously asked, "So are we back to wait and see?"

"No," said Dr. Ribas, "because you are the patient I have been looking for to start a pilot study to justify the larger study. So I propose, if you're willing, to start you on the pilot ASAP."

"ASAP!" the seventy-year-old repeated. "Bring it on!"

As fate would have it, *I* am that seventy-year old and the wife is mine of fifty-two years, Cande. Thirty years on, I ended up chasing the invisible in myself. In this pursuit, I was greatly assisted by the R & D scientists at Ventana, who gave me the critical multiplexed

PD-L1/CD8 results using our third-generation Ventana instrument, even before the tests were commercialized. In the end, I benefited greatly from the company I founded. I received a year of targeted immunotherapy at UCLA under the care of Dr. Ribas. It was an infusion of Keytruda* every three weeks, entailing twenty-one trips to Los Angeles. There were minor side effects, like constant itching, which my dog took to mean I had fleas and needed to go to the vet. The only frightening part of therapy was navigating the San Diego Freeway from LAX to UCLA forty-two times. For that, you had to be well medicated.

In the end, it was my good fortune to receive the latest, best-informed treatment at a critical time, just when medical science had developed immunotherapy to induce self-healing. As always, in medicine—as Tom Weiser well knew—time matters.

This story was tough for Mom. As a parent, to see your son under lethal threat is profoundly unsettling.

But then, as was her wont, she was quick to find a positive in it all. She jumped like a trout on a mayfly with the exciting news that Jimmy Carter, our former US president, was being effectively treated for his metastatic melanoma to the brain and liver with the very same drug, Keytruda*. He was reported to be miraculously responding and, as she said, "So will you."

Mom was to prove prophetic. Four years hence, former president Carter made medical history as he was scan-negative with no evidence of disease in June of 2019.

To the skeptic, it may seem these Nobel-worthy breakthroughs are only available to the elite, to the privileged like Carter, or to a medical insider like myself, but it is important to note that the door was opened to all in May 2018. On that red-letter day, the *New England Journal of Medicine* published a large population-based study including 900 patients with stage III melanoma, showing that the up-front (adjuvant) treatment with Keytruda˚ gave a remarkable improvement in outcome (Eggermont, Alexander M. M., et al., pp. 1789–1801). This impressive study changes the standard of care for aggressive melanoma patients everywhere and ensures that all patients, not just the privileged, should benefit. It also upholds the principle espoused by Dr. Miller that to cure, not just lymphoma but all cancers, you must treat the scan-negative. You must treat the invisible.

Beyond melanoma, immunotherapy is proving highly effective in the treatment of other cancers. And the number of immune blockade drugs is also mushrooming.

A case in point is the recent breakthrough treatment for a lethal form of breast cancer, triple-negative breast cancer (TNBC), with another efficacious immunotherapy drug (anti-PD-L1) TECENTRIQ˚, designed by Roche/Genentech. This breakthrough established a new global standard of care, as it was done in 130 geographic locations in forty-one countries at once (Grady, Denise). This diverse global study was aided by giving all these doctors and all these patients the same state-of-the-art tools. They were all given this latest immunotherapy drug, coupled with the latest chemotherapy agent (nab-paclitaxel from Bristol Myers Squibb), and combined with the latest diagnostic, automated IHC testing done with the Ventana SP142 antibody and the third-generation Ventana instrument.

As it turns out, ten years on, Roche CEO Severin Schwan's vision that medicine should be the same all over the world is coming true—thanks to these new tools.

Epilogue

ONCE BEDRIDDEN, MORIBUND, AND HOSPICE-BOUND, Mom did not die of cancer.

While her multiple cancer sites made the comfort of hospice care logical, she chose instead to fight, to know more, to seek cure. She was not through living.

Her biopsy produced a surprise and dramatically changed her odds. It was a malignancy, but not metastatic breast cancer as suspected, rather a large B-cell lymphoma. The very same lymphoma I had studied and written about for thirty years. The very same lymphoma my wife in Tucson and Beejay in Alaska had faced. The combined therapy that cured Cande and Beejay appears to have cured Mom.

She survived beyond the odds as few ninety-year-olds do. But she was brought to the brink. She had to endure eight months of polypharmacy. She had to bear repeated toxic assault with chemotherapy every three weeks for six months, including two rounds of central nervous system (CNS) infusions. She was subjected to countless infusions and needle pricks. She was made pale, frail, bald, and wobbly. She was dragged to Chernobyl and back. She was left withered and at times an invalid.

Again, she survived beyond the odds. She beat her beast. She was slow to recover, but after a year of hell she was back in the family fold and full of survivor's zeal. At first it was a zeal for simple things, a bit of toast with marmalade, a spot of tea. But no longer bedridden and feeling her strength returning, she came back to one of her reasons to live—her quest to see and hear the rare Trinidad piping guan.

For Mom, the quest to be cured and the quest to go to Trinidad were intertwined. Both were highly improbable and out of scope for a ninety-year-old, but Trinidad fueled the intent and energy needed for an arduous exploit. In a magical way, Mom's inner and outer quests became one—a Holy Grail of health and happiness. It was a pursuit not simply to survive, but to return to vigor and find adventure in far-off exotic places.

Two years on, tramping the broadleaf jungle in the remote highlands of Trinidad, we heard and finally spotted that critically endangered creature. Our pilgrimage was fulfilled with great joy. Now, going on ninety-five at this writing, Mom has realized both impossible quests—the cure and the feathered grail. Both circles are complete.

If we think of cancer as the time thief, one of the great rewards of curing it is capturing more precious time. Curing cancer resets the clock; it turns the dial back, adding precious and unexpected time—and one can do a lot of living in time stolen back.

Mom used every moment to the fullest, and she didn't stop at Trinidad. There was the trip to Mandan Island in New Brunswick, Canada, to see the anchovy-chomping, parrot-billed puffins. There was the field trip to our favorite poet Emily Dickinson's house, her poems read aloud in the car on the road to Amherst. There was the journey to Walden Pond and to Thoreau's woods and cabin. There was Ralph Waldo Emerson's house and Louisa May Alcott's home in Concord. On that day, we were transcendentalists, and we found divinity in nature. We were in turn voyagers to distant lands, birdwatchers, and literary tourists, sharing our common traits of bookishness and curiosity. Along the way, we took the time to talk even more of living in dangerous places in dangerous times, of my brother Tim, and even of thalidomide.

But I was not the only one to share in the richness of Mom's reclaimed life. There was the time spent with her grandchildren, and her granddaughter Emily's wedding in Seattle. There were happy times playing cards and games in the family cottage on the lake in New Hampshire.

At the lake, she began to regale her grandchildren with untold tales. Tales of escaping a murderous mob in Cyprus, of dodging Chicoms in Zanzibar, and skirting green mambas in Liberia. Hearing these remarkable tales, two more generations came to understand they were of adventurous stock—that they should never dilly-dally and always be persistent. These are the extraordinary things that can happen when you outwit the time thief and reset the hands of the clock.

As for Dad, the other half of the universe-needs-improvement equation, after his thirty years in the outfit, and before he passed away, he stepped out of leisurely retirement to drive his own social improvement. Working with some Massachusetts legislators, he drove the creation of a new state law allowing homeownership by the mentally disabled. Specifically, he drove the passage of new legislation that included a special mortgage provision whereby the minimum-hour wages, the HUD assistance, and the Medicaid assistance for the mentally disabled could be combined as collateral for a home loan. The consequence was that my mentally disabled brother, Tim, was the first to own his own condo while on welfare in the great state of Massachusetts.

After affording my brother the enjoyment of living in his own home for years, Tim's condo reverted to the state (by prior agreement) when he passed, thereby returning assets and capital to the welfare system. Dad figured out a way, in true entrepreneurial spirit, to turn welfare into gain. Dad found a way for my brother to live better, while ultimately benefiting the welfare system by returning capital gains. In testament to his social impact, there is today a brass plaque from the Massachusetts legislature commending by acclamation this great achievement now passed on to others.

Today, every time I enter my parents' home in Exeter, New Hampshire, and see that plaque on the wall, I am reminded that the imperative to improve and to take risks was also father-taught.

My other brother, Donald "Buzz" Grogan, was also a part of the family's improvement equation. As a civil environmental engineer, he had an international career during which he spent four years in Egypt cleaning the Nile and six years in Taiwan with his own environmental consulting startup company. In the process, he learned Arabic and Mandarin, making many international friends, and leading his daughters to be globalists who are also contributing to the improvement of the planet.

Dr. Miller became a distinguished internationally known professor oncologist, writing more than 200 scientific papers and living to see his call for chasing the invisible become the standard of care for lymphoma patients after his 1998 publication in the *New England Journal of Medicine*.

JP and Jack Schuler went on to start and fund three more medical companies. JP focused on molecular prediction of cancer treatment response and then on rapid molecular diagnosis of septicemia after he experienced a near fatal blood infection. Both became devoted philanthropists, often giving generously to community education projects.

Staying on one more year after the acquisition, Chris Gleeson moved on to be the chairman of the board (COB) for a medical device company, Genmark, which automated gene testing by a novel method. A few months in, he developed a brain tumor known as an anaplastic glioma with a terrible nine-month life expectancy.

After some Ventana phenotyping and Roche genotyping by PCR, we established that Chris's tumor had the V3 mutation of EGFR (HER1). At the time, there was not a V3-specific drug, but thanks to an ingenious immunotherapy developed by Dr. Henry Friedman at Duke University, Chris's lymphocytes were exposed to a synthetic V3 protein and his newly educated lymphocytes managed to keep the tumor at bay for nearly six years.

Agonizingly, the second unplanned reunion of Ventana soulmates—the first being Tom Weiser's funeral—was Chris's funeral. Again, the faithful flew from all over the globe to salute and lay to rest our beloved master and commander.

In 2019, there was a third reunion of Ventana soulmates, this time planned and joyful. Jim LaFrance, one of the faithful, called for the reunion on the tenth anniversary of the acquisition. That night in Tucson, seeing thirty happy celebrants, I flashed back to the wondrous journey we had all shared. We had all been separated for a decade, but we were still tightly bound together. We had leaned on each other in hard times. This uncommon bond was born of strife and unflinching support of one another.

Among the assembled that night were several who had gone on to either found or head other medical device companies. Jack Phillips, previously our head of sales, became the head of Roche

Diagnostics in North America with several thousand employees. Hany Massarany, who succeeded Chris as CEO of Ventana for two years, became the CEO of Genmark under Chris. TJ Johnson and John Lubniewski, his successor, became CEOs of High Throughput Genomics, a gene expression company listed on NASDAQ. Jim LaFrance became CEO of Omnyx, a digital pathology company and COB of Vermillion, focused on ovarian cancer. Ingo Chakravarty became CEO of Navican, a lab-based genomics business.

Not present that night, but fitting the same mold, were two others. Larry Mehren became CEO of Accelerate, focused on the molecular diagnosis of septicemia and where JP was the COB. Doug Ward became CEO of Personal Genomic Dx, providing genetic testing for pharma.

These eight have gone on to lead their own enterprises with a strongly embedded set of values and well-defined purpose. Their examples affirm that the strongest culture is both transmissible and sustainable.

As for me, after the acquisition, I stayed on with Ventana for nearly ten years, seeing us reach more than a hundred countries as well as seeing us grow the link to pharma and targeted therapies with multiple FDA-approved tests. Eventually, we were reaching nearly twenty million patients and over a billion dollars in revenue per year. Besides this global business success, I was gratified at home, knowing my family, including my wife and mother, had benefited from our technology.

Finally, even closer to home, as the last patient in the storytelling, I have been chasing the invisible within myself. Chasing that last unseen cell, going for cure, was informed by our latest Ventana/Roche multiplex test, processed on our latest third-generation automated instrument, which led to a year of targeted immunotherapy. In that year, after thirty years of practicing medicine, I learned it was easier to be a physician than a patient.

While, nearly four years on, a cure is still possible, it remains uncertain. Even so, there is great satisfaction knowing the fight has been highly informed with a definitive knowledge of the nature of the beast, a well-identified target of therapy, and a matching drug.

As I benefitted from my own and my teams' inventions, I imagined how Edison must have felt at night, reading next to his light bulb.

I know that feeling.

I imagined how he must have felt when he looked out the window to see other homes aglow with his bulbs.

I know that feeling, too.

As for the future of Ventana/Roche Tissue Diagnostics business plan, it remains to be said, it is not just about me, my mom, and my wife. It is about every cancer patient in every hospital, in every city, in every country in the world. Medicine should be the same everywhere for everyone. That's ethical. That's global. So let's press on.

Acknowledgments

MY ACCOMPLISHMENTS IN SCIENCE, MEDICINE, and business were based on strong alliances with others. My method was to persuade others who knew what I didn't know, who had talents different from my own to join in the quest. It took a village to turn an idea into a global company.

I have called attention to a dozen or so of the truly heroic contributors within these stories. But just as important are the additional contributions from colleagues in my lab and department at the University of Arizona, and at the company—both Ventana and Roche.

From my lab at the University of Arizona in Tucson, the key contributors aside from Catherine were two technicians, Yvette Frutiger and Lynne Richter. From the faculty there was Lisa Rimza and Ray Nagle, who were frequent scientific contributors.

At Ventana, there were many who devoted and still devote their working lives to the quest. It is now an organization of 1,400 people, all giving in unison and all deserving great praise for the passionate manner in which they serve patients. I am especially grateful to my administrative coordinator of twenty years, Debbie Mileti, whose ever-reliable and thoughtful support has been an invaluable aid to me and the organization. I owe a special thanks to Hiro Nitta, who so

THOMAS GROGAN, MD 197

aptly ran my lab all these years, and to Kandavel Shanmugam, who has so energetically kept our medical innovation group alive and well and kept us in "blue sky." I am also indebted to Dr. Eric Walk, who has succeeded me as chief medical officer and enabled me to retire with peace of mind. I also owe a great debt of gratitude to Drs. Peter Banks, Michael Lynch, Michael Barnes, Shalini Singh, Patrick Brunhoeber, June Clements, Azita Djalilvand, Monesh Kapadia, Sarah McGinn, Janine Feng, Lupe Manriquez and our other up-and-coming pathologists for their pivotal contributions to our medical departments. All of these MD pathologists are critical to our success as they ensure that as a company we are not just selling instruments and tests but more importantly the practice of medicine.

Critical to our early success were four Ventana employees who were true difference-makers: Tony Hartman, Mike DeGroff, Catherine Wolf, and Bernard Colombo. Tony and Mike were critical to our success at the Cleveland Clinic and many other key accounts. Catherine single-handedly gave us a strong foothold in Europe. First, by establishing a lab and place of business in Strasbourg, France. Second, serving as the chief scientist supporting our expansion through Europe. Bernard was a steady force in our European business, and after the acquisition he was a critical player in the transition to Roche Tissue Diagnostics (RTD), seeing that our Ventana culture continued to flourish.

Special thanks to the cervical cancer team, headed by Ruediger Ridder, Tim Himes, and Jim Ranger-Moore. Also thanks to Pru and Mike Mehta and the Special Stains and manufacturing teams.

I also owe a special thanks to our Ventana and now RTD CEOs. First to Ross Humphreys for giving us a strong start. Then, Victoria Bannister, Hank Petracheck, and Jim Danehy for transforming us into a medical device company. And, of course, Chris Gleeson and his successor, Hany Massarany, for taking us from a product to a market and instilling a world-class set of values and culture. Following them, Mara Aspinall championed our second-generation instruments.

Dan Zabrowski played a key role in connecting us to HQ in Switzerland and driving our culture of quality. After Dan, Ann Costello, coming from Switzerland, oversaw our growth to a billion-dollar-a-year company. Lastly, Jill German, also coming from Switzerland, oversaw our path to world-class manufacturing.

Besides Chuck Hassen, I remain ever grateful to our engineering team, including Kurt Reinhardt, Bill Richards, Wayne Showalter, Chuck Lemme, Kendall Hendrick, Andrew Ghusson and Michael Otter; and to our chemistry team, including Chris Bieniarz and his successors, Jerry Kosmeder and Larry Morrison, for all they contributed.

I will forever be grateful to Dr. Ray Tubbs of the Cleveland Clinic who beyond being a great advisor became a close colleague and friend. He died of a metastatic melanoma before the modern era of immunotherapy. His monumental contributions to Ventana and to the study of HER2 methods is honored every year as the "Raymond Tubbs Keynote Lecture" at our annual Tucson Symposium attended by over 500 cancer doctors and researchers.

Finally, a special thanks to my collaborators who helped me to publish this book: Stacey Forbes, my able assistant who not only transcribed the manuscript but contributed mightily to the creative process. Roman Sandoval, who contributed the artwork, and Marty Hirsch, who has served ably as my reviewer, creative contributor, and publicist.

I am also grateful to Sharon Bially and Emily Adams for their contributions as my publicists.

My thanks also to Stephen Golden, John Smith, MD, Joe Sharkey, Marcus Goodwin, and Emily Grogan, who were insightful reviewers. And Cande Grogan, my first and last reviewer, my inspiration and my partner of fifty-two years. And lastly to John Köehler, my publisher, and Joe Coccaro, my editor at Köehler Books, whose experience and guidance has proven invaluable.

Works Cited

Adams, James Truslow. *The Epic of America*. Boston: Little Brown, 1931.

Dempsey, Martin E., and Ori Brafman. *Radical Inclusion: What the Post-9/11 World Should Have Taught Us about Leadership*. United States: Missionday, 2018.

Durrell, Lawrence. *Bitter Lemons*. London: Faber & Faber, 2009. Page 288.

Eggermont, Alexander M. M., et al. "Adjuvant Pembrolizumab Versus Placebo in Resected Stage III Melanoma." *New England Journal of Medicine*, vol. 378, no. 19, 2018, pp. 1789–1801, doi:10.1056/nejmoa1802357.

Grady, Denise. "Immune-Based Treatment Helps Fight Aggressive Breast Cancer, Study Finds." *The New York Times*, 20 Oct. 2018, www.nytimes.com/2018/10/20/health/breat-cancer-immunotherapy.html.

Miller, Thomas, and Stephen E. Jones. "Chemotherapy of Localized Histiocytic Lymphoma." *The Lancet*, vol. 313, no. 8112, 1979, pp. 358-60, doi:10.1016/s0140-6736(79)92894-0.

Miller, T. P., S. Dahlberg , J. Robert Cassady, Thomas M. Grogan, et. al. "A Randomized Trial Comparing Chemotherapy Alone to Chemotherapy Followed by Radiotherapy for Localized Intermediate and High-Grade Non-Hodgkin Lymphoma." *New England Journal of Medicine*, vol. 339, no. 19, 1998, pp. 21–26.

Smith, Adam. *The Wealth of Nations*. London: J.M. Dent; New York: E.P. Dutton, 1910.

Schmidt, P., et al. "Atezolizumab and Nab-Paclitaxel in Advanced Triple-Negative Breast Cancer." *New England Journal of Medicine*, vol. 379, no. 10, 2018, pp. 2108-21, doi:10.1056/NEJMoa1809615.

Service, Robert W. "The Call of the Wild." *The Spell of the Yukon and other Verses*. Barse & Company: New York, 1916.

Stross, R. *The Wizard of Menlo Park*. Three Rivers Press, New York, 2017, p. 103.

Tumeh, P. C., et al. "PD-L1 Blockade Induces Responses by Inhibiting Adaptive Immune Resistance." *Nature*, 515, 27, Nov. 2014, pp. 568–571.